Reviews

'I have known Cameron Algie for more than forty years. In fact, he was a student in one of my labour law courses in the late 1970s at the Monash University Law School. Cameron has written an extraordinary book on vision loss in all its aspects from the trauma of losing sight, to acceptance, to relationships, employment and even hobbies. He has drawn upon his own experience and on the countless vision impaired persons with whom he has spent time. His clear and cogent style will assist those with vision loss, and of equal importance spouses, partners, children and friends. My blindness occurred at my birth, and I am not aware of any other volume which speaks so clearly to those with vision loss and their families.'
— **Emeritus Professor Ron McCallum AO**, University of Sydney Law School with lived experience of blindness.

'This is an excellent book. I am thoroughly enjoying the read as should be evidenced by how quickly I have progressed in a single morning. 'Overall it was a pleasure to read. Your writing style is lovely - you draw the reader on effortlessly. This should be available for everyone to read. An extensive overview into the world of vision loss. From attitudes surrounding vision loss to the personal, social and societal impacts.'

— **Courtney McKee**, Manager Children and Young People Queensland, Vision Australia. Courtney is a fully registered Psychologist with lived experience of blindness.

"Cameron has done a great job capturing the challenges of vision loss and drawing out the many influences that can impact on the road to acceptance and independence. The book is humorous at times but also sensitive and empathic. It contains lots of practical suggestions and reminders. This book would be a valuable resource for people currently experiencing vision loss, family members, friends, colleagues and professionals working in the field.' It has something to offer us all.'

— **GaryStinchcombe**, BA (Social Sciences) La Trobe University. Dip. Ed. Monash University. Former Deputy Head of RVIB Burwood School For The Blind with lived vision loss experience.
Garry Stinchcombe lost his vision at age 9 and went on to a career in education.

'I loved this book: *I Can See Clearly Now*. I am sure it will be a wonderful guide and help for anyone whose eyesight is deteriorating. Just as important though, it is a tremendous guide for relatives and friends of people losing their sight, and also for those who want to gain an insight into the world of the blind. Of course, it is a devastating diagnosis when you first hear you are going blind but this book is full of great stories from people who dealt with this news and took on the challenges of their fading sight with great courage.

This book is also full of thousands of hints and tricks to live carefully and meaningfully with blindness and for the sighted people who live with them. What I found particularly exciting was how much can be done technically these days for the blind especially with apps for Computers and iPhone. In summary this is a wonderful book I can recommend it to anyone with deteriorating vision and their partners and friends. For someone like me with very little contact with blind people it was literally an eyeopener. A great read.'

Dr Tim Hannah OAM MB BS BSc

This book is also full of thousands of hints and tricks to live carefully and meaningfully with blindness and for the sighted people who live with them. What I found particularly exciting was how much can be done technically these days for the blind especially with apps for Computers and iPhone. In summary this is a wonderful book I can recommend it to anyone with deteriorating vision and their partners and friends. For someone like me with very little contact with blind people it was literally an eyeopener. A great read.'

Dr Tim Hannah OAM MB BS BSc

I Can See Clearly Now

Understanding and Managing Blindness and Vision Loss

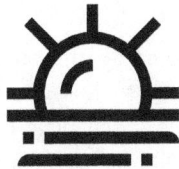

Cameron Algie

AM Ll.B

Facilitator

First published in Australia in 2021 by
Cameron Algie

Cover and page design by WorkingType Studio
Body text & headings: Atkinson Hyperlegible
(https://brailleinstitute.org/freefont)

ISBN:
978-0-6452041-1-7 (paperback)
978-0-6452623-2-2 (hardback)
978-0-6452623-0-8 (ebook)

National Library of Australia

A catalogue record for this
work is available from the
NATIONAL
LIBRARY   National Library of Australia
OF AUSTRALIA

'I can see clearly now the rain has gone.

I can see all the obstacles in my way.

Gone are the dark clouds that made me blind,

It's going to be a bright, bright, sunshiny day!'

Johnny Nash, 1972

Contents

About the Author

Cameron was born and raised in West Gippsland, Victoria, and in the normal course of things, may have gone on to remain a farmer to follow family tradition. However, in the summer of 1968–69, when walking through fields where a full harvest moon hung low, this golden orb suddenly disappeared. Within a few seconds the moon reappeared and there were no clouds in the sky. This mysterious event became the portent of future drama. Cameron was diagnosed to have a degenerative retinal disease with the rather droll name of retinitis pigmentosa (RP), with a prognosis leading to inevitable blindness.

Despite his vision impairment, after studying Law at Monash University, Cameron, became Chief Executive Officer for the industry body representing Cooperative Housing Societies. In his Government Relations and Industry Development role, he created an environment where funding for home loans to this sector grew from $3 million in 1981, to over $680 million nine years later.

During this period, Cameron worked with his wife to establish a Society for RP research. In recognition of this and his Housing Society work, he was made a Member in the Order of Australia in 1993.

Turning back to the Law, Cameron conducted major test cases in nuisance and equitable interests in property, becoming a Member of Planning Panels Victoria, the ministerial advisory body on planning matters.

In a final career change, he later became a Facilitator with Vision Australia where his life experiences and those of clients now form the basis of this book.

Dedication

This book is dedicated as a token of love to my children who bore the brunt of much of my struggles and failures. Likewise, it is dedicated to the many friends, clients and authors with vision impairment, whose stories, tears, laughter, anecdotes and wisdom, makes this book, its messages of hope and practical advice possible. They are and shall remain, torchbearers for change.

Acknowledgments

The writing and publishing of a book doesn't happen on its own. The inspiration of course comes from so many personal and client experiences, the support of family and friends and knowledge that something needs to be put down for the record. I particularly acknowledge and thank the many people with vision impairment whose stories and experiences I have quoted to add so much colour and brightness to the text. I'd like to sincerely thank the following, their order not necessarily in priority, but perhaps chronologically. To my book discussion group, The Mad Skinny Cow Book Club who remained positive and at all times inspirational. To Janene Sadhu for her constant support for my writing, to Sandra Knight for her early critique which headed me in the right direction and Gary Stinchcombe for always being enthusiastic supporters. Susie Barrington deserves a special mention for her courage and capacity to state matters about blindness honestly and for her irrepressible humour so often quoted.

To my editor John Maps of Sydney, whose patience and persistence helped reorganise the book making sense of it all and who displayed so much patience. Also a special thanks to my book designer Luke Harris of Workingtype Studio for his creativity, professionalism and excellence in deciding final format.

Then to others, Dr. Dianne Ashworth, whose friendship I have always admired and treasured, her personal courage and life's story as told in I Spy With My Bionic Eye, told how she was the first woman to act as guinea pig for the Bionic Eye program provided critical early advice and to Courtney McKee who remained a constant friend providing constant encouragement. To my former colleagues at Vision Australia including Ros Chenery and Sarah Taylor who kept urging me on to complete the work. Mention should also be made to Vision Australia for the 14 years of opportunity of working there, after all, it was their long-standing Quality Living Program which provided so much help to clients. Leaders and members of client support groups which flowed out of my Quality Living Discussion Groups always remained encouraging. Fiona Leas, Professor Emeritus David Macmillan Janene Sadhu, and Angelina Piva who carried on the flame of inspiration kindled by groups. Jan Tonkin deserves special mention because of her constant encouragement and wise advice.

Finally, a special mention must go to my family. My sister Merry Bransbury and her husband Geoff, who patiently re-read versions and Geoff who did so much to set up my web site and social media network. My brother Pete and his family also provided inspiration and my sons Hubert and Cameron who remained a constant support and guide on all matters philosophical, motivational and technological.

A special mention and thanks also to Rebecca Karge of the Boroondara Civic Library for her enthusiastic and excellent assistance.

If I have omitted anyone, please accept my apology as it is not possible to embrace everyone who played a part.

Introduction

For over twenty-six years while working as a lawyer and CEO, I lived in constant apprehension, if not all-consuming dread, of making mistakes or failing because of my poor sight brought about by my degenerative genetic condition. Having no central vision, but quite reasonable peripheral sight, I lived in a limbo land, a world of neither being totally blind nor fully sighted, of being detached and yet connected, being complete and yet unfinished.

Sometimes in my legal career, I went to Court so gripped by fear that I became debilitated with diarrhoea and mentally paralysed by fear brought on by nervousness. These insecurities also contributed to a dramatic family breakup in 1999.

While extremely arduous and not to be recommended, this experience actually prepared me well for the fourteen years I was to later spend facilitating client peer support groups for people who were blind or vision impaired. This had the effect of normalising my own loss and allowed me, for the first time, to work without fear of perceived judgement.

As I listened to the many heartfelt and sometimes shocking stories of clients, I worked with them to solve their multifarious vision loss issues. In turn, these stories empowered me to give back to these wonderful people, the insight I gained from them. Retelling their stories explains why so much stigma and nonsense still surrounds vision loss and that there is an ongoing need for greater enlightenment. The many case studies and examples I use in this book are taken from actual one-on-one discussions, but, unless consent has been provided, names have been changed to protect privacy. These stories also come from group discussions with clients and many autobiographical stories with references. Not only do they illustrate the range and depth of feelings experienced, the misconceptions so often found, but they also tell it how it is — a lot of grief, many fears, irrepressible humour, undaunted courage and a compelling story which says that life does not end with sight loss, it is merely the beginning of a new one.

In writing this book it is my hope that these stories — ranging from those of alpha high blind achievers to the experiences of the everyday person with vision loss — will fill a gap in our knowledge surrounding sight loss. People often said they found it too hard to talk about their vision loss with families or friends. As a result, isolation became a common outcome. 'They don't understand me,' 'Take over and won't let me do things,' and 'Don't know what to say and turn away,' were oft-repeated regrets.

In many instances, especially with teenagers, often as a result of peer pressure, they said, 'I don't want to use a computer when my classmates don't.' In this way, isolation becomes a greater issue than blindness itself. Teenagers and many adults refused to face up to vision loss, a response known as 'denial and avoidance'.

In other examples, clients were too fearful of informing

their employers, and unable to tell their boyfriends or families. Extraordinary? Well, yes if you are not exposed to sight loss. However, think for a moment, how would you feel if a doctor said, 'I can't help you; you are going blind.'? Then you are turned out to fend for yourself. Yet, this still happens all too frequently and people are not prepared for the shock of sight loss.

Most people on learning they are to lose their vision, hold deep-seated, yet perfectly natural fears and anxieties, perhaps a strong sense of failure and resulting low self-worth.

With the invisibility of partial sight loss, people say, 'Oh, you don't look blind!' A response which only adds to embarrassment, where withdrawal or disengagement is easier than having to try and explain yourself. Yet, despite the seriousness of this, there is no easily accessible and comprehensive information available in one volume for people who are blind or vision impaired, or for the sighted, on how to face and understand these intense feelings associated with loss of sight, and then gain the practical skills required for leading a successful daily life. This, I felt, is another compelling reason for writing this book.

Approximately one in five Australians has some form of disability. Yet if this is the case, we might expect a broader understanding. According to a recent ABC Media 2019 survey of 54,000 Australians in Australia Talks, it was identified that 75 per cent of respondents said they only 'occasionally, rarely, or never socialize with people with a disability'. Unemployment for people with vision loss is five times greater than their sighted counterparts. So we do have a societal problem worth talking about.

This book provides a comprehensive resource and explanation of the vision loss psyche. I want to show why blindness and vision impairment should not be seen, as is so often the case, as a 'fate worse than death'! While there are approximately 570,000 Australians with some form of vision disability, only 3 per cent are totally 'black' blind. The rest have varying degrees of sight loss. This then surely questions beliefs about blindness. Why is it so feared? Why do others think that once a person is vision impaired they are a liability or useless? How can you respond to the associated loss and grief trauma? What are some of the complete absurdities and humour experienced? What practical tips will allow re-skilling and getting on with a life different to the one you may have lived before?

Also, in preparing this book, chapters are established to be read separately if required, on a topic based approach for easier reference as a resource, or reference book. This approach explains why in some instances, repetition of concepts may occur to reinforce a point.

In answering these questions, I hope to provide a highly readable guide for the blind and vision impaired, their sighted families and friends, professionals, service providers, educators and employers, dispelling much of the misinformation existing about blindness. In the end, to understand that doing things differently is a strength, not weakness and facing up to this is, as with many other disabilities and problems, mostly about attitude.

PART ONE

Insights

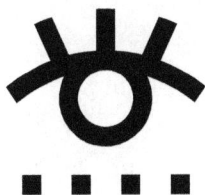

(1)

Blindness and the
Many Faces of Grief

'Those who do not weep, do not see.'

Victor Hugo Les Misérables

'Give sorrow words; the grief that does not speak knits
up the o-er wrought heart and bids it break.'

William Shakespeare, Macbeth.

Blindness is, 'worse than chains, dungeons, or beggary,
or decrepit age.'

John Milton

The Emotional Impacts Of Vision Loss

Losing my sight fifty years ago at a time when I loved reading, relied upon a photographic memory and as an artist, loved light, colour and beauty, was heartbreaking and damned tough, to say the least. At the time vision loss takes place, it can afront the very core of your self-worth. In my own case, I even rejected the love of a good woman, believing no one would want to marry a blind man with no future, a view expressed by other men I was to later meet. In those early days, I felt like Dr Jane Poulson from Canada, who states in her autobiography, 'Nothing could break through the thick layer of anger, fear, loathing and resentment that enveloped me during those dreadful days.'[1]

From 1981 to 2005, I hid the extent of my vision loss, fearful of its impact upon work prospects, or of being judged to be a loser. Like many, I also internalised grief. I used silly excuses when asked to read something, such as 'Oh, I've forgotten my reading glasses!', and by doing so, only perpetuated my struggles. It was many years later, after talking with so many others who reacted similarly, that I found myself somewhat relieved to discover that I was not alone with these inner feelings.

During this time, I encountered misconceptions about vision loss, discrimination, sometimes disbelief, sometimes curiosity and often intrusive requirements to explain my vision impairment. Many people I encountered with vision loss, believing nothing could be done, also thought and said that 'Losing sight was a fate worse than death!' But, on thinking over this latter statement, I began to wonder how could the speaker, not having experienced the latter event, make such a comparison? Death is final, vision loss is not. Nevertheless, it's a commonly held belief. Even the famous blind mountaineer, Erik Weihenmayer, the first and only blind person to climb Mount Everest, said of his early sight loss:

'The fear of blindness had loomed over me for so long and I had never resigned myself to it. It felt like what I imagined dying would feel like and no matter what I felt, what I feared most, this death was coming. . . I had not a clue as to how I would survive as a blind person, how I would cook a meal, walk around, read a book, but trying to live as a sighted person became more painful than blindness could ever be... I also couldn't accept myself as being blind. But one thing I knew, compared to this in-between world, total blindness couldn't be any worse, or any more terrifying.'[2]

Based upon my own experience, I eventually realised that so much about our attitude to vision loss was formed by our perceptions of blindness, the stigma of disability and of how we subjectively interpreted the impact. It was how we thought about these factors which was as great a handicap as any physical manifestations. As Shakespeare said in Hamlet (Act 2 Scene 2), 'For there is nothing either good or bad, but thinking makes it so.' Essentially, as Erik Weihenmayer confirms, when you push through the barriers, you realise it's all about attitude.

However, such loss can never be greater than death. It is actually the shock of lifestyle change brought about by sight loss, our attempts to keep on with our lives as 'normal' and our inability to openly grieve over this loss, that I think we are not prepared for and quite logically, find it difficult to know how to cope with this change. But, it is not all bad. Many people with vision loss I met over fourteen years faced their difficulties with equanimity and general cheerfulness: 'And so hold on when there is nothing in you Except the Will which says to them: Hold on!'[3]

Looking back, I can see clearly now that my initial beliefs were misguided, but then, how was I to know? Now, having undertaken my journey, like Ulysses, survived, re-skilled and gone on to success, my experience has given me a definite advantage when talking to others. The moment I mentioned that 'I've got bad eyesight too!' attitudes of clients changed dramatically, for they felt that someone could understand what they were going through. With this connection I was able to penetrate, then understand, barriers usually thrown up to protect sensitive feelings.

Vision loss, or even partial diminution of this vital sense, arouses such strong feelings of grief and fear that many participants in my group discussions, even those who had been losing their sight for some years, said it was the first time they had been able to talk about it. But why is this so? It is difficult to comprehend that, for many, grief connected with sight loss is as intense as grief associated with the death of a loved one, which explains why people say they would 'rather be dead'. It is after all, the loss of a 'sighted' life which we grieve over. With death of loved ones, however, we are all onlookers and authorised to grieve by society's rituals for mourning. With vision loss there are no such ceremonies or rituals, we may internalise feelings of loss and bear grief for a lifetime. However, positive intervention at an early stage of vision loss can turn this negativity around.

When we realise that vision represents 85 per cent of our sensory capacity,[4] the shock associated with losing so much can be understood. Nevertheless, having to give up work, driving, reading, seeing loved ones and so on, quite naturally, becomes very intense. Many people I spoke with about sudden sight loss said, 'I cried for days!' Or 'I felt my world had come to an end!"

But, as Barbara with age-related macular degeneration (ARMD) in one group said when coming to terms with her loss, 'I may not have good eyesight, but I realise I still have a good brain!' In this succinct way Barbara is correct; there is indeed another life, another way of doing things and we hold other capacities besides vision.

The Range of Responses to Vision Loss

The following client responses from my discussion groups highlight the range of reactions often encountered.

'I haven't told my boyfriend or parents about my Lebers, I am too embarrassed. I just can't bring myself to do it!' (age 32, Lebers)[5]

'I'm afraid to tell my partner how bad my sight is!' (Age 45, Retinitis pigmentosa)

'I was deflated, depressed, I didn't know what the future would be and how fast my eyes would deteriorate.' (age 40, glaucoma)

'It was upsetting, I had a feeling, hoping it wasn't true.' (age 62, age-related macular degeneration, ARMD)

'My family had a history of going blind with glaucoma, but I still couldn't believe it was happening to me!' (age 35, glaucoma)

'When I woke up, I couldn't see and thought what will I do now, I just didn't know what to do.' (age 64, stroke)

'I feel I've lost my identity, my work and all things I knew how to do. I'm feeling angry, sad, what have I done to the world to deserve this?' (age 46, diabetic retinopathy)

'It was emotionally big, I got depressed, couldn't watch TV and went to bed, pushed it all to one side and hoped it would get better.' (age 67, ARMD)

'I thought, Oh grrrr! Now I can't drive!' (age 72, ARMD)

'Yes, It was devastating! I didn't realise my eyes were so bad until I crashed into a train crossing.'
(age 68, glaucoma and ARMD)

'Devastating, I thought I'd received my death certificate, I wanted to die, I thought my life had ended!' (age 43, glaucoma)

Rather than admit disability, many people pretend nothing is wrong. When struggling on day by day gets too hard, they simply withdraw from social life as this appears to be the easiest option. As Gerrard from Victoria, aged 56 with retinitis pigmentosa said, 'I don't go out any more as I can't see in dark venues and there's no hope in picking up a girlfriend! What girl wants to date a person who cannot see? After all, who wants to admit they are disabled?'(See Dating in Chapter13.)

Until we can accept ourselves as now being different, much

of our apprehensions about vision loss, apart from the need to re-skill ourselves and approach tasks differently, is based upon perceptions of what we think others might say or think about us, or the inadequacy arising from not seeing clearly. We may do things differently and feel that we are being judged as fumbling, inadequate, or eccentric. In her book, Blindness for Beginners, Maribel Steel, who has RP, writes, 'There is no doubt that it does take a certain amount of courage to ignore the misguided attitudes you will come across, but what you receive in return for your boldness is good wishes from others who want to support, not judge you. Communicating your truth is liberating in so many ways.'[6]

Grief over vision loss, or reluctance to accept the loss and then tell others, is often not confined to a person directly affected; it extends to partners, families, friends and strangers. As one client reported, 'I couldn't tell my friends, but I later found out they knew something was wrong and they were compensating for this. I found out later that they didn't know what to say, but they offered to pick me up and drive and I felt embarrassed about this!' (age 35, retinal dystrophy).

Indifference and even appalling insensitivity can be commonplace though. One family member said, 'You are going blind, get over it!' In another discussion group, a female client reported that a stranger, on hearing that she was likely to pass on her inherited genetic vision loss to her unborn child, said to her, 'It would have been kinder to abort the baby!'

In navigating this potent brew of complex issues, our feelings are often sublimated. We keep on carrying on with stoic fortitude, 'I won't let this beat me!' This can be both good and bad. Good because, if coupled with anger, it can create determination, perseverance and a desire for action; bad because you might be withdrawing, denying or refusing support willingly offered by others. Or, failing to recognise that technology, re-skilling and another different life is possible.

In most instances, knowledge about availability of supporting services and accessible technology plays an essential role in transitioning to a state of mind we call 'acceptance': accepting our loss of capacity and moving on.

Psychologists now say that 'the process of grieving may differ from one moment to another',[7] so there is no one-size-fits-all approach to understanding vision loss. Everyone's needs are different. It is important to know that a fear of loss of sight can be overcome. Many, many totally blind people say after having lost their sight, 'Life goes on, it's different, but still rewarding.' There is a life after vision loss, and as hard as this may be to believe, we must comprehend this fact if the gap of understanding between the sighted and vision impaired worlds are to be bridged.

Understanding Grief

All clients I met during my Facilitation either had, or were experiencing a sensation of loss and grief. Yet, very few understood the impact this had upon their daily life when these natural feelings were suppressed by a desire to 'fight it,' or 'get over it,' or 'not complain.' It is now accepted by psychologists that grief can lead to greater resilience, if not personal growth, and how we adapt shapes who we become. So, what is grief?

According to the Oxford Dictionary, grief is a feeling of great sadness, unaccountable sadness, intense sorrow.

To understand our pathway to acceptance of vision loss, it is important to comprehend what grief means. Grief is a natural response to loss expressed by sadness, melancholy, withdrawal and crying. It is the emotional feelings one encounters when something like our physical capacities, or someone we love, is taken away. Not being able to see the faces of loved ones, or having a child with vision loss (or other disability) may also create feelings of loss. (See Chapter 14, Parenting.)

Vision loss sometimes comes unexpectedly, with no prior family history, for example through accident. When this happens, shock, self-pity, blame or guilt may be experienced creating barriers to positive rehabilitation.

Feelings of self-pity, blame and guilt can be paralysing in some instances where vision loss is self-inflicted, such as in clients I met who took excessive amounts of quinine,[8] or ignored early signs of diabetes, or in other cases caused by accident, as in one case where a man, playing with explosives, lost all his sight. Many clients with diabetes deeply regretted ignoring early signs and numerous doctors' warnings. As with glaucoma, irreparable damage to the retina can be taking place without you being aware until it's too late. I think many cannot comprehend that diseases that appear so innocuous in their early stages can cause something as dramatic as blindness.

While grief associated with sight loss can be complicated by mixed feelings which make it difficult to stop punishing ourselves, consultant psychiatrist Colin Murray Parkes says, 'Loss is not necessarily harmful and can foster maturity and growth. Grief is a natural process and everyone grieves differently. It can be experienced differently by individuals and be life-changing but we can learn to re-integrate its emotions into our life.'[9]

The process of grieving may also differ according to differences in family attitudes, cultures, character and personality, and we may need to give ourselves permission to grieve in a way that may challenge our customs or beliefs. As psychologist, Associate Professor Christopher Hall Maps notes, 'The focus of coping may differ from one moment to another, from one individual to another, and from one cultural group to another.'[10]

If we accept that there is no exact or correct time for grieving, ongoing sorrow, melancholy, sadness and regrets can take place at any time, leaving us feeling bewildered, out of control and isolated. We can become confused and more forgetful. Elin Williams, [11] a young woman with RP, told the BBC, 'Blindness and mental health will always cause confusion.' At first. Ellen said, 'I felt very lonely and I went through a period of suffering with anxiety and panic attacks as well.' She added that she did not want to go into rooms full of people as this increased her anxiety, a view supported by Professor Ron McCallum in his book, Born at the Right Time 'That the influx of too many sounds and influences can be hard to handle without the filtering, selective process of sight.'[12]

In discussing this adjustment to change, Dr Dean W. Tuttle and Naomi R. Tuttle, who have undertaken research on the impact of going blind, outline a clear adjustment process. Their co-authored book, Self-esteem and Adjusting with Blindness, discusses the process of responding to life's demands and talk about seven stages experienced in developing a new sense of self in rebuilding self-esteem. These stages include trauma response, shock and denial, mourning and withdrawal, succumbing and depression, reassessment and reaffirmation, coping and mobilisation, moving finally to acceptance and regained self-esteem. Current psychological thinking suggests that stages of transition are not sequential and people can move back and forth between these stages. (See Chapter 7, The Psychology of Blindness and Trauma Impact.)

What I often found was that clients find it difficult to express their feelings. They often say, 'No one understands my vision loss!' In any event, it is usually quite difficult to explain what you can and cannot see. This is why peer group therapy is recognised as important in rehabilitation. I discuss such groups later in the book (See Chapter10.).

If participating in a group is not preferred, then writing about how we feel can also release pent-up tension. Elin Williams began to channel her feelings through her blog, which 'helped massively'. Researcher and author Dr James W. Pennebaker, in his book, The Secret Life of Pronouns: What Our Words Say About Us, writes: 'The mere act of translating emotional upheavals into words is consistently associated with improvements in physical and mental health ... those who wrote about trauma evidenced improved physical health. Later studies found that emotional writing boosted immune function, reduced blood pressure and feelings of depression while elevating daily moods.'

Now, at this point let me deal immediately with a typical response — 'I can't write anymore because I can no longer see my computer!' With modern adaptive text reading, or voice recognition technology, this response is untenable, so how about finding out how you can write by consulting service organisations or peer groups? It might be worth noting, that I have not been able to read text or a computer screen for 50 years and use what is called 'text to speech' software. (See also Chapter 18, Technology and Working in the Shed.)

Adjustment Disorder

In working closely over many years with a range of fully sighted service providers, a particular response I commonly heard worried me. Many sighted support staff commonly said that people with vision impairment were 'depressed'. I thought this categorisation too simplistic as in my experience, people weren't depressed, they just didn't know what to do, what technology to ask for, or how to ask for support and so felt no hope that life could be improved. In talking to hundreds of clients, I have only found a mere handful of clients too depressed to consider how to change their lives. The simple fact that reading about what to do, or where to go, being impeded, also restricts capacity to adjust. In most cases, after a short talk highlighting possibilities on how they can keep reading and use technology, the client's attitude became positive. For example, one woman from Queensland in despair over failing eyesight went to immediately download the Seeing AI app. She reported next day, 'Oh, it's fantastic, I've been going around my house reading everything again!' She now leads a support group for people with vision loss.

Once vision loss occurs, the words 'I can't' begin to emerge as a regular statement of presumed fact. This word is accompanied by heightened frustrations, anxiety, anger and a depressive state which of itself, may not mean clinical depression, but rather what is termed an 'adjustment disorder'. This is an emotional low point, sadness or melancholy reached without hope for a cure, future or normality. For medical practitioners, the major concern with this disorder is the duration of this low point and whether therapy, rehabilitation or medication is required. This is also why peer group therapy can be so effective.

As Clinical Psychologist Dr Rob Gordon, psychiatrist and trauma counsellor with the Australian Red Cross states, 'Sadness is not depression. You can learn to manage your sadness.'[13] Dr Gordon says, 'Feelings of grief and loss can have a great effect on your physical health, your mental wellbeing, your financial situation and much more. It is important to acknowledge that these feelings are completely normal.'

From my observation of clients, it is mostly the lack of hope for a solution, isolation and lack of knowledge about what technological and other mobility solutions exist, which contribute to adjustment disorder. Labelling the client as 'depressed' can lead the person away from practical solutions towards medication and negativity. It is therefore imperative that professionals and service providers know:

- about the full range of rehabilitation support services available,
- how peer support groups can 'normalise' loss and lead to acceptance,
- how the range of low and high technology works and what training is available and how this can help,
- how funding or opportunity for support for families can be sourced,

- how to talk with clients so they, in responding, identify their needs. 'I can't' actually offers a solution if you, the practitioner, knows answers.

The Responses of Stoicism and Avoidance

A stoic is a person who endures pain or suffering without showing emotion. The concept of bearing a stiff upper lip is typical of Western culture, and on its face there may be nothing completely wrong with it. However, stoicism connected to disability can become a barrier to rehabilitation.

Like any response to pain, the intense feelings of grief accompanying loss of vision, cause us to pull back — you don't keep your finger in the flame! In all my discussion groups I found that many older people withdraw because it is 'just too hurtful, too bewildering, too hard', or they live with a sense of fatalism. They either didn't know or didn't want to understand that there are alternative ways of doing things to enhance independence.

With stoicism, it is felt safer to keep on in a known comfort zone of familiar surroundings, a response regarded as preferable to change and uncertainty. An illustration of this partial sight loss dilemma, of struggling on using remaining sight rather than adopting other alternatives, is provided by Bill, a client with macular degeneration. He complained, 'My eyesight has got worse over the years and I can't read the aisle signs in supermarkets. Why can't they make the print on these signs larger?' Yes, this question sounds reasonable, but practically speaking, how large must these signs be made to suit everyone? Bill's response is typical of so many who have not adjusted fully to their vision loss and attempt to keep functioning in a sighted world. In effect he is asking, 'Why doesn't the world adjust for me?'

Bill went on to say that he thought he'd adjusted to low vision, advising that he had a smart phone yet didn't know of several options available that would enhance his smart phone use and improve his independence. For example, he could use:

- smart phone apps such as Seeing AI, which will instantaneously read these signs in the smallest of fonts
- assistance provided by a supermarket's Customer Service Desk, where staff will willingly assist
- use free apps provided by supermarkets which provide information, such as which aisle a product is in, contents and price (this depends on whether you can recognise items on the shelves)
- supports provided by other agencies or volunteers
- online shopping and home delivery.

In a state of stoicism our emotions are suppressed with well-worn clichés, such as 'I must keep a stiff upper lip!' Or, 'Grownups don't cry!' Or 'I'm OK, I can manage!' Or, 'Oh, don't worry about me dear, there is someone worse off than me!' 'My mother never cried and I was brought up not to show emotions.' Or as a survivor of recent bushfires in Victoria said, 'You've just got to pull your socks up and get on with it!'[14]

Yet the impact of suppressing our emotions may be accompanied by ill health, loss of appetite or headaches, as well as further feelings of self-doubt, embarrassment or guilt which further inhibit us.

We don't like admitting to our disability. The thoughts 'What if?' Or 'If only!' or 'I wish!' come flooding in, indicating regret and lack of acceptance. These responses show that a person is still wishing for a return to the past, or a quick fix. Buddhist and other philosophies say, you cannot change what has gone before, only the present, so negative responses to sight loss only act to put off the inevitable.

What is required is a reality check, a recognition of what is actually happening and that there may be no immediate cure. This honesty leads to acceptance — an acknowledgment of who I now am and getting on with life's activities again. As writer Sheri S. Tepper says, 'Nothing limits intelligence more than ignorance; nothing fosters ignorance more than one's own opinions; nothing strengthens opinions more than refusing to look at reality.'[15]

Making yourself busy is often used as a way of getting on with things. Oh stop thinking about yourself! Just get on with it! This can be helpful as a distractor, but as a form of putting things off, psychologist Hugh Mackay says, 'Making yourself busy is a trap, a hiding place which appears legitimate, but actually avoids reality.'[16]

Talking about Vision Loss

Another dimension of the problem of withdrawal is evidenced by a consensus of views expressed in peer group discussions. It is that vision loss brings about an unwillingness to talk about it, which may have many causes. We might see ourselves as a failure, or be shy with low self-esteem.

On the other hand, it is genuinely not easy to explain poor vision to others. Your vision may be blurred, you still can see, but not clearly. Your vision may vary throughout the day, or be worse at night. We may find it irritating to keep responding to unhelpful but well-meaning questions such as, 'How much can you see?' Or, 'Won't new glasses help?' Or 'Why don't you try medications, or health products?'

Generally speaking, we may feel overwhelmed, we find ourselves in a new territory with which we are unfamiliar, and with no certainty or famly patterns providing comfort. This experience is well paraphrased by ABC broadcaster Leigh Sales, who states in her book Any Ordinary Day, 'The brain relies on searching for familiar patterns to help settle on an explanation with which we feel comfortable.' She says, 'This is influenced by three things, past personal experience, evolutionary biology and the experiences of others. What were once real fears have now disappeared or have been internalised into our belief system. Threats become terrifying when you don't know how to prepare a response.'[17]

Why Re-skilling Is Important in Dealing with Grief

Through my own personal experience and through observation of others I have come to understand that if a person with sight loss can re-skill themselves, they can maintain work, sustain families, and regain independence, hope and confidence. If this cannot be accomplished early in their vision loss trajectory, then they will most likely remain for too long in a shadow, if not grip, of grief. The ideal is to achieve a balance between avoidance and confrontation, which enables the person gradually to learn new skills, come to terms with, then 'let go' of the loss as circumstances change. Perhaps as sight diminishes slowly, we may need to revisit these responses regularly.

In the midst of all these feelings, it is worth reflecting that we did not learn how to be blind at school. In many respects, as we now need to re-skill ourselves to function differently to the way we did before, we simply may not be emotionally ready or equipped with skills for what lies ahead. Now, with vision loss we need to, in effect, 'go back to Grade One', to re-skill ourselves, learn to do things differently, to start life all over again.

Initially, there will be disbelief and incredulity when told, 'You do not have to see things to do them.' With our natural impulse to look at things, this is hard to accept. Now technology can restore our capacity to function, a positive fact virtually non-existent ten years ago. With this understanding, we can now move on.

(2)

Impact, Types, Causes and Effects of Vision Loss

'A blind man knows he cannot see, and is glad to be led, though it be by a dog; but he that is blind in his understanding, which is the worst blindness of all, believes he sees as the best, and scorns a guide.'

Samuel Butler, 19th century novelist

'To be blind is not miserable; not to be able to bear blindness, that is miserable.'

John Milton, 17th century poet

There are hundreds of books and articles about eye conditions, and this book does not attempt to be a medical authority. However, in this chapter I have summarised eye conditions most frequently encountered during my discussion groups to assist with an understanding of what most clients experience. A short explanation on their causes and effects is provided.

How Many People Are Blind?

There are an estimated 253 million people with vision impairment in the world today. Approximately eighteen per cent of the blindness diaspora are regarded as Legally Blind (a status deserving government support with a pension), but may still have some useable sight. The vast majority of people with vision impairment, approximately 79 per cent, have varying degrees of vision impairment. There are about 575,000 people in Australia, over 28 million in the USA and many worldwide who experience degrees of vision loss, not total blindness. (Of the world wide figure, approximately half have correctable sight.)

While untreated eye conditions such as uncorrected refractive errors[18] form the largest cause of vision loss worldwide and are usually treatable, in Australia, Europe, the USA and other 'wealthy' countries, the most common causes of sight loss are:

- cataracts, causing cloudiness, blurredness and loss of colour
- age-related macular degeneration (ARMD), causing blurredness, sometimes bleeding and loss of focusing ability
- glaucoma, causing pressure affecting the optic nerve; it is incurable but can be controlled with eye drops or surgery
- diabetic retinopathy, caused by diabetes, causing blurredness and bleeding can receive treatment.

All can lead to legal blindness and some to total blindness. However, control of blood sugar levels with diabetes, anti-VEGF therapy injections to prevent bleeding with wet macular degeneration[19] and eye drops to reduce pressure for glaucoma, plus constant monitoring, are required.[20] Most of the above have genetic origins.[21]

Vision loss is most associated with age. Even without eye disease, people aged eighty years will probably need approximately four times more light than a twenty-year-old as vitreous fluid inside our eyes, initially crystal clear, becomes discoloured by advancing age. This process means you require more light to see and explains why many older people ask for brighter light to see things clearly.

Older people experience a higher proportion of sight loss than the rest of the population. Cataracts amount to 40 per cent and macular degeneration to 28 per cent of vision loss in older Australians.[22] Yet there are many causes of vision loss that can have far greater impact on sight.[23]

In Australia, approximately 66,000 people (approximately 11 per cent of those with vision impairment) are classified as 'legally blind'.[24] That is, their vision loss is so advanced that they qualify for government benefits and pensions. These numbers are expected to double by 2024 as the population ages.[25]

Some Causes of Total Blindness

In my discussion groups it was quite common to encounter people with cancer of the retina (retinoblastoma), tumours on the optic nerve,[26] retinal detachment, or industrial and motor accidents as causes of total blindness where intense shock and trauma is experienced. Up to the mid-1960s, a common cause of total vision loss was the oversupply of oxygen to premature babies, called retinopathy of prematurity (ROP, formerly called retrolental fibroplasia). Too much oxygen damages immature retinal cells. In these cases, the baby's eyes, but for this oversupply of oxygen, may have been normal had the baby survived adding to feelings of parental guilt.

Children can be born with congenital (meaning 'at birth') eye conditions such as cataracts, Detached Retinas, or early macular degeneration (called Stargardt's disease), or anophthalmia, a condition in which one or both of the baby's eyes do not form in pregnancy. In these cases the brain's visual cortex receives no or little stimulus, and this is known as amblyopia.

Early sight loss affects development of the visual cortex (the occipital lobe), the primary cortical region of our brain. The main purpose of the visual cortex is to receive, segment and integrate visual information, which is subsequently sent to other regions of the brain to be analysed and used. This process is highly specialised and allows for the brain to quickly recognise objects and patterns without a significant conscious effort.[27]

If neuro pathways and the visual cortex of the brain do not develop as they do for people with sight, those blind from birth may have what is emotively called 'black blindness'. This effect has been described as just a 'black space', 'a nothing'. On the other hand, Helen Keller had what she called 'white blindness', suggesting some early stimulus of the visual cortex had taken place before she lost her sight at the age of nineteen months from what was thought to be either meningitis or scarlet fever.

If there is no cognitive state of vision, the brain does not function. There are no images of colour or form, although comments from people blind from birth say these images can be 'learned and a sixth sense develops'. For example, Professor

Ron McCallum, blind from birth with ROP, in his book *Born at the Right Time*, talks about his perceptions of colour: for him, the colour blue is an ocean made up of 'sounds or feelings; salt, wind, sound and sensations', which are of course not 'blue' at all... grass which we all know as green is for Ron, 'soft, spikey, short, spongey or squelchy.' Ron says, 'I had to learn to live with the limitations of not truly understanding the whole content and context of the world around me, colour, proportionality and visual description continued to have different meanings compared to those with sight. I have always found it difficult to describe people in visual terms, even those I know well. If I am honest I would struggle to describe our children's appearances.'[28]

Ron says the big things 'like driving a car or seeing a sunset are not annoying 'I don't quite understand that!', but the little things, says Ron, like 'dropping and losing things are annoying'. He says that major differences are more 'sensual, aural, tactile and smell whereas for those with vision, its visual, like looking at a map.'

It is therefore important for sighted people to understand that, for the vast majority, (approximately 79 per cent)[29] of people with vision impairment, varying degrees of sight are still experienced. These people are not totally blind, but have vision impairment ranging from mere light and dark perception, such as knowing it is daylight or night-time, to minor blurredness, with parts of the peripheral field seeing clearly, as in macular degeneration, or with quite clear quadrants of sight as in the effects of stroke. With these groups, visual images are retained, which provides both a powerful emotional impact of loss and a retained memory to 'see' things. This is the category of 'blindness' which causes most confusion for sighted people. Blindness can be partial, so please don't assume the word blind means blackness. (See Chapter 6.)

Charles Bonnet Syndrome

This topic is worth discussing here as in many instances, people with low vision experience vivid images of, houses, gardens, faces or swirling, flashing lights. These images make some believe they are going mad. One peer support group member, Margaret from New South Wales, described this effect well when she said, 'I was walking down the street and saw a brick wall and I stopped as I thought I was about to crash into it. But it suddenly disappeared!' In another group, two participants said that, because of their agitation over the effect of these images, they received Community Treatment Orders and were admitted as involuntary patients in psychiatric institutions.

These visual hallucinations are known as Charles Bonnet Syndrome (CBS), which is similar to the phantom limb syndrome, an effect in which the brain retains memory after amputation of a leg, still feeling toes that are no longer there etc.[30] However, with CBS, no pain is normally experienced.

People born totally blind do not normally experience CBS, which makes sense because the visual cortex is not stimulated. The syndrome mostly affects older people who lose sight later in life from conditions such as macular degeneration. Although professionals are not exactly sure what causes CBS. it may be related to visual memory fragments encoded in the brain's visual networks.

There are some coping strategies for CBS sufferers:

- Avoid sensory deprivation and sedentary lifestyle, i.e. go outside and receive greater visual stimulation.
- Strengthen social contact and physical activity.
- Undertake purposeful eye roaming (scanning) or extended eye closure techniques.
- Optimise vision if possible by surgery (for example, for cataracts) or medicines.[31]

A Positive Future, Technology and Medical Research

Many people who are totally blind retain their independence by using technology to buy food, clothes, services and travel online.

When vision loss occurs at a later age, habits and confidence established up until that point are often shattered. Older people may not want to identify with blindness, or associate with the blind community and may prefer to wait for their doctor to find a cure or treatment. In using smartphones for example, to trust that, with built-in speech, you do not have to see the phone to use it, remains a constant point of incredulity. On the other hand, making it work for you, apart from the usual frustration, remains a moment of great exhilaration. (See Chapter 18, Technology and Working in the Shed.)

With today's technology, many of the former barriers have fallen away, and the opportunity for participation in study, work and the community has never been better. However, the fact that less than 25 per cent of blind or vision impaired people have full-time employment appears to suggest that stigma, fear, perhaps poor preparation and discrimination in the workplace still remain potent factors.[32]

With the introduction of latest artificial Intelligence (AI) technology over the past ten years, many fears of vision loss — and definitely the boogeyman, that once blind you are useless — can now be dispelled altogether. Text to speech audio technology enables those with vision loss to participate in work and maintain independence. Voice recognition technology is now revolutionising the ability to participate in the workplace and home. Self-drive cars, the bionic eye and treatments or even cures using stem cell or gene therapy are being developed.

There is already successful gene therapy treatment for hereditary eye diseases such as Leber's optic amorosis and choroideremia. Moorfield's Eye Hospital in England has successfully grown stem cells to form new macular cells in trials for people with 'wet' macular degeneration. But while those with disabilities await these results and affordable treatment, how we face vision loss and lead full lives is the challenge I will deal with in subsequent chapters.

3

Coming to Terms with Vision Loss

'Blindness is not the barrier; it is the attitude of the "seeing" which is the barrier.'

Helen Keller

'Sometimes, I feel I am really blessed to be blind because I probably would not last a minute if I were able to see things.'

Stevie Wonder

The Mixed Messages of Blindness

Helen Keller overcame both blindness and deafness, and became famous for her activism, writing, travel and achievements. She disproves the idea that life is finished or of no value if sight is lost. Importantly, apart from her own perseverance,

Helen benefited from the patient teaching of Anne Sullivan so that Helen became the first blind person to earn a Bachelor of Arts degree. It wasn't easy, though, as due to her early unruly behaviour, family members thought she should be institutionalised. Her mother thought differently, never gave up and constantly sought solutions. Helen's story however, highlights a major theme of this book, that perseverance, asking for help and relying upon others to assist where necessary are key factors for a pathway to success.

Of course, the impact of sudden vision loss cannot be dismissed lightly. Dr Jane Poulson, who lost her sight in her late twenties due to type 1 diabetes writes, 'I was terrified, I suddenly felt very vulnerable. When my bandages were removed, my disappointment was palpable ... desperately I clawed at the invisible band over my eyes. . . Blindness was very close to a lethal blow for my self-esteem and my sense of myself as a medical professional. A stroke of a surgeon's scalpel snatched all this away from me!'[33] Yet, despite this pessimism, Jane went on to practise as a totally blind doctor until her death in 2001. She relied upon friends and colleagues to assist, for example, in the observational diagnosis of a patient's condition.

Yet surprisingly, when we think of all the fears of blindness, anomalies remain, presenting mixed messages. We value the statue of Blind Justice as a symbol of impartiality, so as not to treat friends differently from strangers, or rich people better than the poor, so what's wrong with that? Blindness is seen as an advantage. Love is also blind, meaning all forms of human frailty can be overlooked by feelings of love — nothing wrong with that either! As William Shakespeare said in A Midsummer Night's

Dream, 'Love looks not with the eyes, but with the mind, And therefore is winged Cupid painted blind.'

People who are totally blind achieve worldwide fame for their accomplishments –nothing weird about that either, as there are no supernatural powers accompanying blindness although historically, people superstitiously thought so. But discrimination in the workplace and community still exist, along with false perceptions about blindness. For example, a recent Scientific American article continued the folklore of 'blindness' by referring to highly developed sensory skills of the blind as 'super powers'.[34]

In reality, increased sensory and perceptive capacities often attributed to people who are blind are no more than our brain's natural ability to rewire itself (neuro-plasticity), in which neuron pathways grow thicker and stronger with increased use, like muscles. With blind people, the visual cortex can be used to improve hearing, touch and other senses.[35] This also explains why echo-location can be successfully used and why heightened senses are possible. This is not super-human or supernatural; it is a power available to all of us. When exercised, neuro-plasticity merely further illustrates our amazing human potential.

According to researcher Corinna Bauer, 'The brains of people blind from birth, or who lose sight later in life, make new connections to boost hearing, smell, touch and even cognitive functions such as memory and language. Structural, functional and anatomical differences in the brains of blind people are not present in normally sighted people.'[36]

Generally speaking, blindness is not a barrier to life and achievement. Fear of blindness and attitudes towards disability are barriers enough.

What Is Sight?

We live in a world dominated by sight. Vision is the process of deriving meaning from what is seen. It is complex, learned and a developed set of functions that involves a multitude of skills.[37] Our sense of vision represents about 85 per cent of our perception, learning, cognition and activities, which are mediated through vision arriving at an appropriate motor or cognitive response.[38]

We have highly developed vision called 'stereoscopy', that is, seeing in three dimensions to give us special depth awareness. We are also brought up to identify others by the way they look, and much emphasis is placed upon reading these signs, especially in work or social environments where body language is regarded as important. Nevertheless, we can function without sight. Our sense of hearing, taste, smell and touch are, of course, important, and they will become even more so when we lose our sight as a result of the brain's neuro-plasticity.[39]

After all, as already noted, we are not dealing with an insignificant problem. According to the World Health Organisation (WHO) 2019,[40] and the medical journal Lancet,[41] numbers of people in the world with blindness and low vision are expected to rise to 550 million by 2050, largely due to ageing populations.[42]

Fear of Darkness Also Leads to Fear of Blindness

Many people, both young and old, hold fears of the night and darkness. So much of sight is connected with our worldly orientation, and we probably all have fears of becoming lost in the dark, or of night blindness, which can also be a medical condition.[43] Fears of associated dangers, such as crime and fear for our safety, are logically connected. These negative images of darkness and blindness are often portrayed in literature and movies, reinforcing these fears. For example, in H.G. Wells' The Time Machine, the Morlocks are ape-like creatures who live underground in darkness like blind moles and are repelled by light. They surface only at night to devour innocent Eloi, childlike humans, and this plays upon our subliminal fears of darkness intertwined with moral forces of good and evil.

The film Silence of the Lambs also plays on our fear of being blind. In one terrifying scene set in a pitch dark cellar, sighted Detective Clarice Starling has to find and shoot the villain, who has the advantage of night vision glasses. We all imagine the terror we might feel if placed in this situation. However, even current presentation of blindness in literature and film continues false concepts of vision impaired people holding supernatural powers or skills.

An example of this nonsense is the popular 1995 film, Scent of a Woman, with Al Pacino, where a depressed, blind retired army officer can, with little or no guidance from his sighted friend, among other skills, drive a car through the city at breakneck speed, unscathed. Really?

Words also Portray Blindness as Negative

Many terms, verbs, adjectives and nouns portray negative images we associate with blindness. Examples include 'blind drunk', 'blind as a mole', 'blindsided', 'blind as a bat' and 'blind folly'. Such terms mostly use blindness with gloomy effect. They suggest incapacity of some sort, being caught unawares, or without hope of redemption. These terms and others all contribute to our pessimistic perceptions of blindness as a disability.

If we think about it, fear of blindness stems as far back to the cradle of civilisation. Ancient Egyptian and Greek mythology and Biblical references all create indelible and mostly negative imagery of blindness as punishment for wrong-doing. Negative attitudes towards blindness have been evident for centuries, transitioning into literature, cinema and culture in general. For example, in Robert Louis Stevenson's 1883 Classic, Treasure Island, Blind Pew the pirate is characterised as hapless, shouting for help, cursing and wildly tapping his stick while on his way to the Admiral Benbow Inn. This fearful image of blindness is expanded through the portrait expressed by young Jim Hawkins: 'I never saw in my life a more dreadful looking creature ... this eyeless creature!' It's an image that may also help to strike fear and loathing in our minds about blindness.

But is blindness really that bad? Michelle Hackman, a blind US journalist has this to say: 'Blindness is not a life-threatening disease — for many, not even a condition significant enough to stunt personal success. Yet sight is so essential to the concept of living that people feel some sort of an existential attachment to it, as if to lose their sight would be akin to losing life altogether.'[44]

It seems also appropriate to reflect that most prejudices, for instance, xenophobia or racism, exist because of a lack of knowledge — ignorance about another land or people's culture. With blindness, lack of knowledge about what people with blindness can actually achieve supports a stigma and fear of this disability. Ignorance may be bliss, but to use an old adage in this case perhaps makes the point: 'None are so blind as those who cannot see.'

Dialogue in the Dark

The 'folk tales' of blindness created by literature and pseudo-scientific mumbo jumbo could also be finally overturned by expositions such as Dialogue in the Dark, created by Andreas Heinecke in Frankfurt, Germany, in 1988. After the premiere, Heinecke toured the exhibition worldwide, and there have been more than 130 showings in 30 countries.

The main concept of the exhibition is a role reversal, where in a totally darkened room, blind people lead sighted people around. Those with sight are torn from familiar comfort zones, losing, as I have noted previously, what is their primary sense: sight. In this way, sighted people's inability to comprehend what vision loss and blindness really mean can be overturned. It is very much a practical experience, requiring both parties to depend on their 'available' senses, something that literature and films simply cannot do.

Developing other Skills

In his autobiography, blind Professor Ron McCallum writes about the differences in senses between the blind and not blind, saying that the 'major differences are more sensual, aural, tactile and smell, whereas for those with vision, it's visual. Development of early aural skills is critical for speaking and communicating … a critical advantage in society'. Also essential is touch, says Ron. 'My fingers are in a real sense, my eyes. Touch has its own security.'[45]

In addition to Michael Hingson who, in his book Thunder Dog, described how he developed echo-location skills, Daniel Kish from the USA, who has been blind since he was a baby, is able to use a human version of echo-location by making a series of clicks and noticing changes in their 'echo,' to 'see' the world around him. Others, such as Ron McCallum and Susie Barrington of Sydney, say they can use their sixth sense to 'see' people in a room. 'I know someone is there and my son gets surprised when I say, is that you?' says Ron.

Everyone may have at some stage closed their eyes and wondered how they would cope experiencing loss of horizon, not seeing, then groping for a landmark, plus fear of falling, becoming disorientated or lost. It is vital to understand that all these apprehensions can be overcome by re-training ourselves to do things differently. (Further details on practical tips are discussed in Part 3.)

Many of the sighted person's fears of blindness may also be based on false assumptions. For many people with sight, a white cane means someone is lost, or that it is a 'symbol of the stigma of disability', rather than understanding as Steve Kelley of the USA says, that a white cane actually is an 'important navigational tool.' Apart from detecting changes to the pavement, a cane also provides additional 'sound' identification. It is often assumed that white cane users are totally blind, but this is not so. (This is discussed further in Chapter 17, Orientation and Mobility.) But, it's also important to know that many people with vision loss can manage well without using a cane.

Hearing what vision-impaired people say about blindness reveals that misconceptions can be overcome. 'To suggest that there is no reason to feel anxious or fearful to someone experiencing vision loss would be inaccurate and insensitive,' writes Steve Kelley. 'A visual impairment will bring changes to their lives, profound challenges at times, moments of intense frustration, and ultimately the determination to relearn those tasks we all take for granted — like getting to the grocery store or reading print. It is not an easy transition, but it can be managed so much more effectively with less of the cultural stigma and fear many of us hold about blindness.'[46]

Some High Achievers

We are all amazed by what people who are totally blind accomplish. We must remember that at the heart of their achievement, they are just ordinary people who persevere. In the face of enormous adversity, blind activists such as Tilly Aston in Australia, activists Joseph Campbell of England and US activist Professor Dr Jacobus tenBroek, founder of the National Federation of the Blind (NFB) and equal opportunity activist Haben Girma, the first deaf-blind graduate of Harvard Law School, successfully overcame seemingly insuperable odds usually created by sighted people.[47] Erik Weihenmayer, a totally blind mountaineer not only climbed Mount Everest but also the other six tallest mountains of each continent.[48]

Dr Kenneth Jernigan (longtime leader of the American National Federation of the Blind, NFB), represented the blind and vision-impaired community in promoting the right of those with vision disability to be listened to in setting national disability policies and not have these policies dictated by sighted leaders of service delivery organisations.

Other political activists include Juan Carlos González Leiva of Cuba and Sabriye Tenberken of Germany, co-founders of Braille Without Borders. Australians such as marathon runner and adventurer Nick Gleeson, marathon runner Gerard Gossans (also noted for his participation in the TV show Dancing with the Stars), Professors Ron McCallum, Professor Laurie McCredie, legally blind artist Alan Constable and blind writer and poet Barbara Blackman, are also notable.

These people are but a few who demonstrate what those who are totally blind can accomplish.

Yes, even blind people become medical practitioners. Against the odds, Jane Poulson, author of The Doctor Will Not See You Now, had a successful career as a doctor, despite being blind. Transcending her anger, fear, shock and denial at her vision loss, she travelled to northern Quebec to undertake medical work for the Inuit people, and also travelled to France, Bermuda and England. She used colleagues and friends to describe what her eyes could not see. In addition to medicine, she took part in cross-country skiing, swimming and water-skiing. Phew! Don't you feel exhausted? Another world beater was the American Francis Salerno, MD, Geriatrician from Philadelphia, blinded by type 1 diabetes. The first blind internist certified by the American Board of Internal Medicine, he was named Clinician and Physician of the Year by professional bodies.

Blind sportspeople and adventurers have achieved incredible things. Going back to the nineteenth century, James Holman – known as the 'Blind Traveller' — travelled extensively in Europe and throughout the world. Much more recently, in the 1990s, Miles Hilton-Barber — British traveller and climber — sailed solo from Africa to Australia.

Among other blind high achievers are Ugandan-Norwegian athlete Tofiri Kibuuka, one of the first three blind people to reach the summit of Mount Kilimanjaro, and British Member of Parliament David Blunkett, who served as a minister under Prime Minister Tony Blair.

Surely these stories tell us that disability through blindness is not a barrier to success. Then what is? Is it, as Helen Keller says, attitude?' Michael Hingson of the USA, would agree. Michael, who with his dog guide, survived the 9/11 Trade Tower collapse, says that it is how we believe in ourselves, which is the answer.[49]

Other People with Blindness Also Lead Successful Lives.

High achievers are one thing, but many quite ordinary people with vision loss also maintain happy and productive lives. They keep their independence, work for a living, study to further their careers, and take part in sport. Barry in Queensland, who is totally blind, is a parachutist. How does Barry do this? He doesn't dive tandem, but with a friend who jumps after him and uses a radio to give directions — another example of reliance upon friends to achieve what you want.

Michael Simpson, from New South Wales, is the former State Manager for a national vision agency. As a boy, he lost one eye as a result of playing Cowboys and Indians with bows and arrows. Later as a teenager while working at his father's service station, in a second fluke accident, someone in a passing car shot at him with an air gun, blinding him in the remaining eye. Michael said, 'Losing my sight was a shock, it was terrible at first. However, with hindsight, I think it was the best thing that happened. I went to Sydney and learnt how to live a different life. I learnt that I had a whole lot of skills I didn't know existed. I think my life in the world of vision impairment has been much richer as a result!'[50]

Janet Shaw, from Western Australia, is another who kept on despite the odds. She lost an eye to retinoblastoma (eye cancer) when young, but after treatment retained some sight in one eye. However, aged thirty-three, her remaining eye gave way to cancer and she became totally blind. In her book, Beyond the Red Door, Janet writes about how she sincerely believed that she could not live if her sight were to completely fail. However, despite her blindness, Janet rose to win several world records as a tandem cyclist.[51] Again, Janet relied upon others to become successful.

Sue-Ellen Lovett, from New South Wales, is a totally blind champion horse rider, who has competed in dressage events in the equestrian Paralympics and represented Australia many times since 1994. She also raises money for Guide Dogs. How does she do it? 'I used to get lost in the arena a lot with my horse "Desi" and he used to shy a bit,' she says. 'I think he was testing me out — "if I do this again she'll give up on me" — and that was scary. But I just had to tell myself to put my big girl pants on and be brave. All through my life, my guide dogs and horses have allowed me to be just like everyone else.' In recent times she too uses others to assist her, like calling out arena numbers as guidance. 'I'll keep riding and competing for as long as I can. I hope I'm proof that you can do whatever you want to do — you just have to find a way,'[52] perhaps making the point again, that how we manage vision loss is all about attitudes.

Empathy, Not Pity Is Needed

In conducting my discussion groups over fourteen years, one response that I found clients universally loathed, was when pity was expressed such as, 'Oh, you poor thing!' Or, 'I'm sorry you are blind!' (See further discussion on this point in Chapters 5 and 6.) The sighted attitude also shows itself when sighted people are too embarrassed to inform a blind person that something might be not working, or is wrong.

From a sighted person's point of view, what are better attitudes to adopt? It is empathy, not sympathy that is required. However, empathy is the least used of our natural responses. Empathy comes from an understanding, of 'being in the shoes' of someone else's experience. Susie Barrington from Sydney, who lost her sight from a tumour on her optic nerve, experiences situations where, when walking with her dog guide, strangers come up and offer sympathy to her by saying, 'Oh, I'm sorry you are blind!', to which Susie responds, 'Why? It wasn't your fault!'

Why are we so pitying of disability and blindness in particular? Is it our lack of contact with disability generally as the ABC radio survey showed? Is it our lack of understanding of what we can accomplish with vision impairment? Or pity based upon these apprehensions? Or our innate, ingrained fear that sight loss and its presumed darkness makes us vulnerable, helpless and hopeless? Is it an assumption that blindness means you need protection, or that you must go into a 'home'? Or that once blinded, life is finished? Probably all of the above, and we shall consider these in detail in subsequent chapters and why they are misplaced.

It stands to reason, therefore, that if we have very little to do with people having vision loss, or for that matter, other disabilities, then we will also have little understanding, tolerance and empathy for this world and how those with vision impairment actually fit in. This is the barrier — or should it be the challenge for fully sighted people to understand, and for workplaces and institutions to accept.

Perhaps the last word in this Chapter should go to Mike Hingson, who with his dog guide Roselle, survived the 9/11 World Trade Center disaster. Mike escaped down seventy-eight flights of stairs with Roselle beside him unfazed by the calamity. 'We must not let fear paralyse us, we must carry on ... to build a better society through trust and teamwork, and we can make it happen!'[53]

4

Some Aspects of Communicating with the Blind

'Wisdom cannot be imparted. Wisdom that a wise man attempts to impart always sounds like foolishness to someone else ... knowledge can be communicated, but not wisdom. One can find it, live it, do wonders through it, but one cannot communicate and teach it.'

Hermann Hesse, writer and Nobel Prize winner

'Self-consciousness kills communication.'

Rick Steves, writer and TV personality

Explaining Vision Loss to Others

While at university with no central vision, there was still no need to use a cane for mobility, so there was really no need to disclose my disability until I absolutely had to. So for me as with many thousands of other people with partial sight, vision loss can be a hidden disability. In the University library, once finding a book, by peering closely, nose brushing a page, I could see large print, book titles , sometimes even decipher page numbers, or if font was large enough, chapter or case headings, but that was all! So, I approached students with book in hand and asked, 'Could you help me read this? I am Legally Blind.'

The dumbfounded student would look at me, think I was joking, turn away and walk off without saying anything. I soon learned that to use the term 'blind', when to all extents I did not look so, caused confusion. Instead, I learnt to ask, 'Oh, can you assist me? I have bad eyesight.'

The results were astounding, most people could identify with this experience and understand. Often they said, 'Yes, I've got bad eyesight too, I must get new spectacles!', then would quite happily proceed to assist me.

With communications, assertiveness skills are important. Claudia, from New South Wales, displayed excellent assertiveness when she said, 'I just told my neighbours that I couldn't see very well and that if they wanted to talk to me to first give their names. They all do now and it makes a real difference!' Yet few people with vision loss possess this degree of confidence and assertiveness.

Using terms that do not confuse others is important in any field, but where emotion and stigma is attached, it's doubly important. For example, in my university anecdote, saying I was Legally Blind was accurate, but it confused people because I still retained some sight and did not need to use a cane or ID badge — I did not 'look blind!' As discussed in the last Chapter, the word 'blind' carries a powerful negative message, while on the other hand, sighted people do understand what low vision or bad eyesight means.

How Sighted People React to Vision Loss

To maintain a healthy perspective on this subject, I need to state that not all those experiencing sight loss are negative, nor are reactions of sighted friends and strangers necessarily unhelpful. However, there is a significant gap between these two poles — the sighted and the blind — which leads to misunderstandings and some humour.

One factor I constantly observe is that sighted people are afraid of blindness (perhaps disability generally?), or don't know what to say or how to offer to help. For example, Graeme Innes, former Australian Disability Discrimination Commissioner, tells the story of how he, a totally blind man, was admonished by an unknown woman while standing on a Sydney railway station, for having his young child with him on the platform. She demanded his name and said, 'People like you should be reported !' Presumeably believing a blind man incapable of looking after children and on a dangerous train platform too! In response, Graeme threatened to bring a case for harassment. [54] Did she really believe Graham could not look after his children? Laughable? Well, yes, at a distance, but not at the time when such comments catch you off guard and if you are still adjusting to vision loss, challenging your confidence.

Strangers can react in ways that surprise, bewilder or hurt us. Their responses can also add to our frustration, anxiety or stress. Some responses as reported in my group discussions included:

'Friends ignored us as though the problem did not exist.'

'Friends took over without asking and grasped my hand to lead me, not guide me.' (See the explanation of sighted guide techniques in Chapter, 17 Orientation and Mobility.)

'My children assumed I am incapable of looking after myself and want me to go into an aged care home.'

'They expressed disbelief and intolerance towards me and said, "You are putting it on!"'

Another facet of human contact was where my group participants reported sighted people were often inclined to speak louder to someone with vision loss, as if they were also deaf. Alternatively, rather than asking the person with vision impairment directly, they asked a partner, 'What does she/he want?' In some instances, small change from a payment made by a person with vision loss would be placed into the hand of the sighted companion. Why? Do sighted people really believe someone who is blind is also incapable? This behaviour all seems so nonsensical. Joy Thomas, in writing for the Vision Aware magazine on this problem says, 'As part of the sighted person's inability to understand how others cope with vision loss, they often raise their voices as if hearing were a problem, assume intellectual capacity is diminished by speaking in simplistic terms, intervene offering to help without finding out first whether you need help.'[55]

In another example, Bill from Victoria, a seventy-five-year-old pensioner said, 'The cleaner is driving me crazy. She keeps moving things around and I can't find them. Even when I tell her not to move things, she doesn't take any notice.' I recommended that he try simulation glasses and get the cleaner to use them, after which Bill reported, 'She always puts things back now!'

(Simulation glasses, made from cardboard with a plastic lens, mimic certain eye conditions to convey the visual effect of an eye disease and can be quite helpful in conveying what is hard to explain about vision loss.)

Fears of Blindness Confirmed

Results of research conducted in 2014 by the American Foundation for the Blind (AFB) provides some answers as to why reactions to blindness are so irrational. This survey confirmed that most people deeply fear blindness, although many might say that death and cancer are greater fears. Of those who participated in the survey, 62 per cent said that the loss of vision was the single most frightening possibility they would ever have to face. Nearly 88 per cent of people surveyed, considered having 20/20 vision vital to good overall health, while 47 per cent believed that losing their sight would have the gravest effect on their daily lives. Loss of independence and quality of life were the top concerns for respondents. Over 60 per cent were aware of common eye conditions like cataracts and glaucoma,[56] while other AFB research identified, 'Losing vision would be as bad as, or worse than losing hearing, memory, speech, or a limb.'[57] One can begin to understand fears associated with blindness support a widespread stigma that blindness is a disability to be avoided. It is usually an uncertainty of what to say, perhaps stemming from shyness or politeness, which also underlies this problem.

Is there a Special Language?

Sadly, but factually, there are people who fear blindness and respond as though sight loss means you are helpless, hopeless, deaf, dim-witted and no longer possessing capacity, or faculties to do anything. My own experience and that of many in my groups, is that sighted people are afraid to ask, 'Do you have useable sight?' or 'Do you need some assistance?' Or perhaps they feel that correcting a person with vision impairment, if they are clearly making mistakes, is insensitive or hurtful.(See Chapter 6.)

I also found many vision impaired people became uncomfortable with using normal 'sighted' terms such as 'reading a book' or seeing a movie. This attitude stems from a sort of honesty we have in describing what we are doing.

These 'normal' terms also confuse sighted people who become unsure about what is polite or 'politically correct'. They often apologise, 'Oh, I'm sorry! I didn't mean to say that as you can't see.' But why be embarrassed? Does it really matter if blind people continue to use words sighted people take for granted and make communication easy? No, not at all! There is no need to feel awkward or create a special language.

In support of the above proposition, Rosemary Mahoney in The New York Times, 2016, said, 'Friends have told me that, before they met me, they wouldn't have known how to communicate with a real blind person, as though there exists some separate language or code of conduct governing our interactions.'[58]

A common experience is when sighted people do not know how to speak to you when eye contact is non-existent, or someone is using a white cane. Mary, with diabetic retinopathy in Victoria, said, 'Why do the sighted always ask my partner what I want — tea or coffee and not ask me?' Do people with blindness speak another language? To refer to Joy Thomas again:

'Just because our vision changes doesn't mean our interests do. Some people assume that certain hobbies that are sight-related, such as sports, fashion, makeup, woodworking, etc., are no longer interesting or feasible after vision loss. This simply isn't true. There's nothing worse than a group of friends assuming that you no longer want to go on your annual bike-riding trip, aren't interested in watching a football game together, or don't enjoy shopping with them anymore. Yes, some things may change, such as needing to use a tandem bicycle or a tether for running side-by-side or audio descriptions for movies, but these activities can still be very fun. There are always ways to compensate and adapt when it comes to the activities we love.'[59]

Another factor to keep in mind is that people with sight may feel embarrassed about telling you something is wrong, for example that your shirt is dirty or that an article of clothing is inside out. In her book, *The Doctor Will Not See You Now*, Dr Jane Poulson told of how, when handwriting a patient's notes following their admission to hospital at 2am, that she had been writing for half an hour when a colleague doctor came over and 'told me that my pen had no ink. A nurse who had been sitting nearby for all this time burst into tears and said that she didn't know how to tell me, that she was afraid of hurting my feelings'. Jane said, 'Next time just say that my pen is not writing! I would never be angry with them If they pointed out my mistake.'

In a not too dissimilar example, Susie Barrington from Sydney with her dog guide 'Tilly,' told of how, one day in the supermarket, the customer service lady said, 'Oh, You are so inspiring!' 'Why?' asked Susie. 'Because, well,' the lady hesitated, 'Well; You do all these amazing things ...', hesitating again.

'Why, because I'm blind?' the indomitable Susie interposed, correctly guessing the lady couldn't say, 'Because you are blind.'

Slightly embarrassed, the customer service lady said, 'Well, yes! Because you're blind!'

It was so difficult to say that mysterious word 'blind', and we have to ask, why is this so?

However, Susie in her inimitable way got the best out of this situation by using humour. She went on to say to the lady, 'Well, if my dog guide wasn't so dumb she could do all these things for me and I wouldn't have to!' Susie continued, 'Anyway, Tilly's too young to cross the road by herself, she's only six!'

It does pay to see the humour in things.

The adventurer Erik Weihenmayer, in his book 'Touch The Top Of The World' says, 'One of the false assumptions surrounding blindness was illustrated by a lady too afraid to use the word "blind", when she asked, "How long have you been a person of sightlessness?" Maybe she thought that blindness was a kind of demon and just the mere mention of the word blind might give it the power to rise up and crush my spirit.'[69]

For those with vision loss, normal communication skills adopted using eye contact and body language are challenged, to say the least.

However, people born blind who have received careful schooling, report that if they were taught to focus on a person's voice, they could look the speaker in the face. The Jolley and Gleeson families in Victoria say the same, and Dr Jane Poulson also trained herself after losing her sight as a result of Type 1 diabetes, to 'look at the voice'.

Sighted people sometimes have a tendency to push, grab or pull people with vision impairment without first asking 'Do you need help?' or 'Can I assist you?'

In a US National Federation of the Blind (NFB) article, Barbara Cheadle points out that, 'As social rules about touching are taken seriously, they are seen as part of our individual freedom, we expect that rules for touching with strangers, family, teachers and carers, for sighted people also applies for people who are blind or who have vision loss.' It would seem reasonable to assume that the same social standards regarding touch should apply equally to the blind. 'Too many sighted people, on seeing a blind person,' says Barbara, 'rush to offer help on the assumption it is needed.'[61]

Understanding Medical Jargon

There are so many types of partial vision loss that the term 'blind' itself could be a misnomer. The term 'partial sight' or 'vision impaired' would seem more inclusive. (Note: Many sighted people refer to those who are partially sighted as 'visually' impaired. 'Visually' is an adverb meaning 'related to appearance', for example, when someone is inspecting a road. Calling someone 'visually impaired' suggests they don't look too good!) This terminology appears to be so entrenched it is incapable of changing, but my personal plea is to stop saying 'visually impaired'. As mentioned above, only 3 per cent of those with vision loss are totally black blind; 18 per cent who are functionally blind may still retain some 'useable' sight and the rest with partial vision can often see well enough to maintain mobility and read, albeit slowly.

Apart from inexact use of English, perhaps part of the problem in our general communications about blindness is the mystique of medical jargon surrounding eye disease. Medical terms, often based on Latin or Greek, might be convenient shorthand for medicos, but they can be confusing for the lay person and help keep doctors in a pre-eminent position.

To the lay person, a medical diagnosis may sound complex, perhaps mind-numbingly perplexing. Nevertheless, it is definitely my view that in coming to terms with vision loss, it remains important for the ordinary person to understand what their eye condition means and for doctors to realise the impact of their diagnosis and explain impact in lay terms. If unclear, the person affected, their partner or family member needs to demand and obtain answers from their medical adviser. If nervous or worried that you might forget, place your questions in writing, or bring a friend or family member to the appointment, who, being less likely to be stressed, can take notes, seek further explanation and also be able to listen to and then explain objectively later, what has taken place.

I frequently hear about people being reticent to ask their eye doctor about their diagnosis. I am a great believer, that when in doubt, obtain a second opinion, even if this means going outside the public hospital service. One client from South Australia with glaucoma reported that, in the public hospital, not only did doctors change with each appointment — leading to confusion as to what was wrong — but that the incessant chatter of orthoptists in charge of eye tests, distracted her concentration. It was lucky that she followed my suggestion to see a private specialist, who then advised she must urgently change her medications. She rang six months later to thank me, because the specialist had advised, she said, 'Had I not changed medications, I would have lost my sight!'

The following are the most common causes of vision loss:

Stroke can cause partial loss in segments or quadrants where one half or three-quarters of sight can be lost, a condition called hemianopsia. The remaining segment can retain clear vision.

Cataracts (the most common cause of vision loss in both wealthy and third world countries) creates loss of acuity, fogginess and glare. In most cases, replacing the opaque lens resolves sight.

Glaucoma and diabetic retinopathy create patchy, darkened and blurred vision, often leading to total sight loss if neglected. Many clients coming into my discussion groups deeply regretted ignoring doctors' warnings connected with early stages of diabetes and glaucoma. Diabetic retinopathy is the largest cause of blindness in people of working age.

Age-related macular degeneration (ARMD or MD), which leads to central vision loss, can still leave useable peripheral vision for many years. There are two types, wet and dry. Wet MD, so named because of bleeding in the retina, can be treated by injections. Dry MD has no bleeding with a mottled appearance in the retina caused by buildup of small yellow or white spots called Drusen. A healthy diet and lifestyle and some supplements are usually suggested.

Retinitis pigmentosa, a 'dystrophy' or degeneration of retinal cells caused by genetic defects, normally causes tunnel vision with peripheral field loss, but some atypical cases have the reverse effect with central sight loss.

Genetic disorder has three types of transmission: dominant, affecting all within a family; recessive, with a 50 per cent chance of offspring becoming affected; and X-linked recessive, where the faulty gene is transmitted to offspring via female carriers, although recent information suggests a 2 per cent probability women will also be affected, with a 50 per cent chance of inheritance. Affected families should obtain genetic counselling.

Scared as Hell, but I Must Go On!

I think the main reason why most people are so afraid of blindness is because of the tremendous lack of awareness about different ways to cope with vision loss. Organisations like the Chicago Lighthouse Foundation, American Printing House for the Blind (APH), the Royal National Institute for the Blind (RNIB) in Britain, and blindness agencies in Australia such as Guide Dogs and Vision Australia, Canada and New Zealand and other countries, offer a wide array of programs, services, training and technologies which allow people with varying levels of vision loss to remain successfully independent.

'As hard as it might be to believe for those newly diagnosed with sight loss,' says the Chicago Lighthouse Foundation, 'most fears and misconceptions about blindness and vision impairments are surmountable. Losing one's sight does not have fatal consequences.'[62]

Fear is part of our DNA and is not confined to blindness. When Professor Jacob Bronowski was making his Ascent of Man series for television, a plane the TV crew were using in the African Rift Valley crashed on take-off. The next day Jacob asked the pilot,

'Are you OK to fly with the other plane?' The pilot replied, 'Well, I'm as scared as hell, but I know I must go on!' This was the message used in this series, that mankind in facing challenges might be as 'scared as hell' but we still push ourselves onwards. And that, 'My dearly beloved', as Rudyard Kipling would say to his readers in Just So Stories, is what people with blindness and vision loss also do!

(5)

Dealing with Families and Friends

'Research shows that perfectionism hampers success. In fact, it's often the path to depression, anxiety, addiction, and life paralysis.'

Professor Dr Brené Brown, social worker, author,
lecturer

'My dear young cousin, if there's one thing I've learned over the eons, it's that you can't give up on your family, no matter how tempting they make it.'
Rick Riordan, author and teacher

Typical Family Responses

Perhaps not unsurprisingly, families present one of the most complex scenarios for people experiencing vision loss. Blindness raises the sorts of hard-to-articulate apprehensions I've discussed in earlier chapters, while others in the family may see those with vision loss still functioning normally, leading to disbelief, that there is nothing wrong. For example, 'Mum carrying out her daily tasks doesn't look any different!' Or, 'Dad, in complaining about difficulties in seeing things, is only exaggerating!' On the other hand, those with vision loss may also hold an unreasonable expectation that other family members will naturally understand what they are going through.

There are many examples of a partner or family member being overprotective, worrying about safety, or feeling inadequate in knowing what to do with the vision-impaired person's slow physical responses, for example, they might step in and take over, or hold back. Friends or family might want to assist, but find it easier to take over as it is quicker and there won't be such a mess, for example, while cooking in the kitchen. However, well-meaning help can be disempowering and confidence-sapping. In one group, a lady with macular degeneration who had lost confidence after her husband had taken over cooking duties, was jubilant when she returned to the kitchen to make a casserole after five years of 'exile'. 'I made a mess,' she happily reported. 'But I did it!'

Creeping into this admix of responses is a perception that, partial sight loss as with Macular Degeneration, means you are also incapable of continuing. Many become frozen; 'I can't see therefore I can't!' become the operative thought processes. All this is unnecessary of course, for we can re-skill ourselves to do things another ways.

In one group, Maggie from Queensland, who had severe diabetes and vision impairment and was also an amputee, was at her wits end with a husband who didn't listen. While he liked preparing food for the household, he controlled the pantry and fridge, which suited him, but his arrangements were inaccessible for Maggie, who couldn't read normal print and felt frustrated, locked out and angry. I formed a view that the husband's dominance was based largely upon his view that his wife was over-emotional, but in any event, he liked cooking and preferred taking over this task. When the husband came to her group, we were able to let him see how upset Maggie was, recognise the importance of her participation in cooking, then discuss some strategies so that he would agree to work with her. They needed to organise both pantry and fridge so that Maggie could find and access products on her terms, not his.

While some women may be only too pleased to give up chores of cooking and housekeeping, for many, as in Maggie's case, the loss and grief experienced in becoming excluded from their main role in the home, can be soul destroying where loss of vision is seen as the primary reason. Similar feelings are expressed by men who find themselves excluded from their work, workshop or working with machinery. A number of group participants said that their well-meaning partners had thought using machinery too dangerous. One man advising of his devestation when his wife insisted he 'sell' all his wonderful power tools. This approach is completely unwarranted as a safe set-up can be organized to make working safe. (See Chapter 18 Technology and Working in the Shed.)

Much anguish is also expressed by wives who try to retain a perfect household, but feel they cannot do so. Issues such as dusting and cleaning general household mess create high levels of stress. Joanne from New South Wales, with MD and who later became a peer volunteer supporting client groups, said, 'In the early stages of my MD, I tried to keep on going, entertaining friends, but one day while trying to organise a party, I just broke down, I realised I couldn't keep on pretending nothing was wrong. I had to tell my friends what was happening and then I found what I was worrying about didn't matter, they were all supportive!'

Sometimes using the wrong ingredients may cause embarrassment, for example, 'I found the cat food wasn't all that tasty!' said one group participant. 'I made gravy out of my cup of tea and wondered why it was a bit wishy washy!' said another. These mishaps become comical when one is not so stressed about these mistakes.

A sensible point expressed by many peers with vision impairment who support discussion groups, is, 'Well, if you can't see the dust or disorder, it doesn't matter!' If it worries you, arrange for cleaning support. Others say, 'Well, when my sister/ friend comes over and says, there's dust on your furniture, I give them a rag and say, please wipe it down then!' For those who are house proud, it can be a great relief to realise that you don't have to worry about so much detail when others are there to assist.

Peer discussion groups also reveal there may be ethnic and cultural barriers hindering acceptance and independence. In an Italian family, the wife said, 'My husband refuses to let me use the white cane at all!' In another group where a strong Greek patriarch ruled, a wife was not permitted to keep in touch with an ongoing telephone support group. The wife's disappointed response was 'My husband won't let me take calls from other members of our group, I'm sorry!' In other groups where participants were from Asian or Middle Eastern backgrounds, while strong social or church networks existed to provide support, the stigma of blindness remained so strong that clients were over-protected to the point where they saw themselves as helpless.

In other families, a disbelief around the virtues of technology can apply: 'Oh she doesn't need all those gadgets, or that new-fangled smartphone!' This attitude stems from a lack of understanding of how much modern technology can really assist with independence. In one family, the totally blind wife was continually told by her husband, who was himself vision impaired, that she 'did not need an iPhone' because he himself did not need one, and could therefore not see how benefits of an audio-based phone, GPS and other voice-driven or voice-activated apps could assist. As a result of group discussions, she bought an iPhone, which she now says is the best thing she ever did.

While confidence can be lost in the early stages of sight loss, a partner may also be reluctant to accept that change is necessary because they, too, are unwilling to accept change, or face disability. Rather than stepping in to 'solve' the problem, it is more helpful if a partner or family member approaches the difficulty presented with vision loss by, understanding that re-skilling by the partner with vision loss is essential, and asking, 'How can I help you?' In talking to a partner, be prepared for an answer that might be, 'Oh, I'm OK dear!' The typical stoic's response.

Coupled with the above tendency to take over, is making yourself busy as a form of avoidance and claiming that you have all the answers as a form of denial. Dianna Seybold, an outstanding Facilitator in Victoria, pointed out these characteristics when in her group, a woman kept telling the others how she 'solved' everything concerning her Macular Degeneration. I asked Di why was she in the group as she appeared to be coping. To my surprise, Di's response was, 'Wait and see, she hasn't adjusted to her vision loss yet!' This turned out to be correct as in session six, the woman broke down to admit how terrified she was and yes, didn't want to admit she couldn't cope, or accept her disability.

A family member wishing to assist needs patience to listen; let the person with vision loss work through their needs and then work with them to devise organisational systems and strategies which work. Importantly as a sighted partner, do not presume that because you can see it, she or he can. In my groups I have seen this latter point occur again and again, where a partner with excellent sight just cannot understand what partial sight really means so that a degree of intolerance is present. In these instances, simulation glasses, which mimic the effect of sight loss, are essential. (See Chapter 16, Independence in the Home, for practical tips.)

Grandparents and Children

Many grandparents with vision impairment reported their upset and grief that their children will no longer leave grandchildren with them. 'I am so upset that my daughter will not leave her children with me anymore and I can't seem to reassure her that it will be all right!' Is an oft repeated complaint. There is a natural and powerful desire of all parents to protect their children of course. The sighted child's fears, albeit genuine, that 'Gran' won't be able to see if something (usually unspecified) goes wrong, may make them afraid to let grandparents mind their children. This has happened in my personal case as well as to many others. Patience and education are required in these circumstances. The issue is, are these fears justified or are they based on lack of knowledge, or mere assumptions? Often, emotions flowing with vision loss are so upsetting they contribute to an inability to articulate clearly how you, the grandparent, can manage safely, adding to the child's grief and uncertainty. After a lifetime of child raising you, as a grandparent, will surely believe in your child-minding skills. But it is worth remembering, if totally blind parents successfully raise children — and there are many instances of this, there is no reason why people with partial sight cannot undertake this role. (See Chapters 14 and 15, Parenting and School Issues.) While parents feel their proven skills in child raising are being completely ignored, it may be that their children think otherwise. That parents 'didn't do such a good job in child raising anyway!'

One vision-impaired woman with macular degeneration reported on her success. 'I got my daughter to stay with me for two hours at a time and then a little longer each week so that she could observe and I could demonstrate I could manage OK,' she said. 'Eventually she consented that I could have the child overnight, then the weekend. It was a matter of understanding and trust, I think, when she could see I would be OK!'

A further commonly expressed grief of grandparents with vision loss is, 'Oh, I feel so bad that I can no longer see my grandchildren and read bed-time stories anymore!' Well, do we need to stress? There are several options here. While the loss arising from not seeing faces, reading books and watching children grow is genuine, heartfelt and not to be dismissed lightly, there are still other ways of communicating.

We can still touch and talk to children, play games using large print or tactile games and, above all, listen — a skill that will clearly convey emotions. One group leader uses simulation glasses to play hide and seek where her grandchildren using these glasses, try to find others. 'They keep asking to play this game and now want their younger sister to also play with 'Nanny's' glasses!' she said.

If the child is old enough, they may describe their school day, a picture or even read a book to you, allowing you to embellish the story. This is definitely beneficial for the child's reading skills. Or you can tell stories of your childhood or life that are usually well received. Some people with vision loss who are skilled Braille users like Graeme Innes, quite happily read aloud to their children as their fingers can follow the story.[63]

Young children have an amazing capacity to accept disability. Children are not inhibited, as adults can be, by prejudice or social values. Often grandparents explain their vision loss by saying, 'Gran has 'broken' eyes!', and children will quite happily read to become 'Gran's eyes' and be 'Gran's little helper' with walking and shopping. This support gives a child a natural sense of self-worth and pride in contributing to a family member they love unconditionally, although this may wear off by teenage years.

A mother with vision impairment wrote:

'At this young age, Claire (sighted) learned that I watched over her by using a combination of tactile methods as well as keeping up a constant chatter to know what she was doing ... I encouraged my daughter to come to me at regular intervals, and tried to turn my dependence on her visual assistance into a game of hide and seek ... My children loved to be Mummy's eyes, and would run to help me find a missing sock, a misplaced earring or inform me on the activities of their siblings — except on some days when they were more inclined to disregard my requests in favour of their natural need to play.'[64]

If it is your grandchild who has vision loss, there are excellent tactile books from Vision Australia's Feelix Library, which will allow you to share a book with young children.[65]

Alternatively, a great range of children's audio books is available in Public Libraries, or commercially.

Smother Love and Learned Helplessness

A person's capacity to respond to vision loss may also depend upon existing domestic roles played within a family unit. Where one partner has been largely dependent upon the other, for example for cooking, washing and house care, actual, learned or acquired helplessness may exist even prior to vision loss. In recent discussion groups, Bill from Victoria and John from Queensland both wanted to do more around the home to reinforce their own feelings of independence, but they both expressed their frustration as, 'My wife does everything and I find I am simply not allowed to play a role.' This highlights again, the need for assertiveness and a clear understanding that vision loss does not prevent you from retaining skills.

On a similar theme, James from Victoria with macular degeneration had a wife who refused to let him intrude into her domain. When she went away on holidays, James found himself truly helpless. 'I couldn't cook or even use the washing machine.' In desperation he said that he'd resolved to go into respite care. On hearing his stress, I arranged for an Occupational Therapist

(OT) to urgently attend his home and quickly set up his systems with tactile markers, little sticky pads he could feel. Suddenly James found he could successfully carry on with household duties, and his frustration levels subsided. However, upon his wife's return, to his disappointment, like Bill and John above, James was once again precluded from undertaking household roles. Clearly, if a greater participation is desired, some re-negotiation of roles is required. This can be formalised with help of family counsellors, Orientation and Mobility instructers, or Occupational Therapists.

From another point of view, other family members, thinking you incapable of looking after yourself, say, 'You should get a cane, get a dog, get new glasses, or go into a home!' etc. These terms have the additional effect of disempowerment, taking away your capacity to look after yourself. (See Chapter 6, Things that Disempower Us) In fact, this attitude can foster over-dependency, leading to learned helplessness.

The widespread belief which assumes that once you have vision loss, you are incapable of doing anything, is worsened by the shock reaction experienced when losing sight. As Erik Weihenmayer said in his book, *Touch the Top of the World*, 'Ironically, as I relinquished my grip on sight, I sank into bitter relief. I had not a clue as to how I would survive as a blind person, how I would cook a meal, walk around, read a book, but trying to live as a sighted person became more painful than blindness could ever be.'[66]

If there is any plea to make, it is for those with sight not to take over, not to assume blindness means helplessness, not to step in feeling sorry, but to ask what assistance may be helpful and find out what tasks are possible, remembering that re-skilling, the capacity to undertake tasks differently, is a key understanding for sighted carers. Always encourage re-training for the person with vision impairment; it's never too late. I have seen people in their nineties and even a man of a hundred years, re-skilling themselves with technology so they can use their Internet and remain independent.

Sighted carers also need to be aware that, particularly among an older generation, a blind person is not helpless or hopeless. One lady aged 94, was protesting about changing to Smart phones. At one point I asked her, 'What did you do in the past?' 'Oh, I managed 90 staff!' she responded. I then said, 'Well, do not try and tell me you havn't got the personal capacity to learn how to use modern technology!' Within the next month, she had purchased an Iphone, a phone plan and agreed to undertake technology training.

In their early life, many clients may have been managers and leaders. Invariably when I contacted older aged clients by telephone, partners said, 'Oh, Fred just sits in his chair all day and listens to the radio!' Or 'Bill is afraid to go out on his own so I have to always walk with him!' Or 'I have to answer the phone for John because he can't see it!' are typical, but completely unhelpful family situations. (assuming of course, no other disability is the barrier.) Every person has different vision needs, and if this is how a family chooses to live, fine! But, it is important for a carer to understand that such dependency is not caused by vision loss.

A carer may also not find it easy to create time for their own personal 'self-care' space if they feel committed to look after a helpless 'blind' partner. 'Jack can't see and keeps asking me to read to him, or do things for him!' said one exhausted carer. But, why should this be so? There is now, as mentioned, an enormous range of low-cost reading, audio devices and personal training available. There are many mobility supports and occupational therapy skills training available through blindness agencies to increase independence and confidence. There are volunteers who assist with walking, cycling and other activities. It is important these services be taken up when sight loss begins. Finding out who can help and then contacting your local blindness agency, is a practical first step. Doing so will head off a natural defence of stoicism, or anxiety, or 'I'm too old to learn!' usually proffered as an excuse for not taking up training or supports.

There may also be some fear of change and reluctance to accept disability included in responses. A carer needs to know these solutions exist and be firm for their own sake as much as the person with vision loss. It is surely the carer's duty to encourage independence rather than dependency. Support, including financial support, is available through Carer's organizations, or support bodies, along with government programs providing Carer Allowances.

Typical Family Responses to Blindness

We may not realise that family members can be apprehensive or even fearful of not knowing what to do or say in dealing with vision loss and this only adds to unhelpful responses. If the vision loss was caused by a genetic problem, other family members may even have fears that they too will inherit. A woman from New South Wales said that her parents from two differing European cultures argued vehemently with each other as to 'whose faulty genes' created her vision loss. 'It was quite vicious and it really upset me and I felt it was my fault they argued!'

A mother from Victoria said recently, 'My son is angry and unhelpful with me. When I was at the airport, he said, "Why are you using your stick? And why are you looking up into the air like that?" I said, "Well, I'm trying to find the red guide rope so I can hold on and also trying to see how far it is to the end of the reception hall!" I don't think he accepts my vision loss; he doesn't like me using my cane and I think he hates it and is in denial!' As previously discussed, use of simulation glasses, or education of her family using Orientation and Mobility Specialists, could bring about an understanding of what vision loss means.

However, with late onset of vision loss for a parent, teenagers can be particularly awkward, rebellious and rude. One mother from Queensland said: 'My fourteen-year-old daughter gets embarrassed if I use the cane and asks me not to use it. She says that she'll help by holding my arm, but that she didn't like me using the cane!' Some people give their cane a name and even decorate it, treating it as their best friend — a way to get their cane to be accepted.

Changing Roles and Relationships

The vision loss story is multifaceted, for example a sighted partner may have difficulty adjusting to the effects of vision loss on the other partner. In one Victorian family an angry and frustrated wife said to the husband, 'You don't know what it's like living with vision loss!' To which the weary and frazzled husband responded, 'And you don't know what it's like living with a person whose got vision loss!'

If communication in the relationship has not been strong in

the first place, vision loss could well be a trigger for relationship breakdown. In one group, a client reported, 'I lost my job, my wife left me and now I've lost my home!' In some instances, angry, aggressive or destructive behaviour, such as heavy drinking, can contribute to marital breakdown, and it is too easy just to blame blindness for this behaviour.

Quite surprisingly, partners say they are reluctant or embarrassed to admit to their partner they have vision loss. 'I was too afraid to tell my husband!' advised one forty-five-year-old client with a genetic eye disease. 'But my husband didn't assist me and I had to work on him for ten years!' was the response of another weary wife from Victoria, who lost her sight slowly with retinitis pigmentosa. One woman from New South Wales with glaucoma said, 'My children are fine and help me, but my husband doesn't help me at all. He keeps holding my hand and I don't find this helpful and when I ask to hold his arm, he doesn't seem to understand, or want to cooperate. Either he doesn't accept that I'm no longer the independent person I was, or he is unwilling to assist! He's interested in other things like sports, but not wanting to assist me now!'

Many believe their partner will reject them. This fear is not unjustified as I've encountered a number of cases where a partner with vision loss had been deserted. Dianne Ashworth with retinitis pigmentosa, describes in her book, I Spy With My Bionic Eye, how her husband could not cope; he eventually left her nearly blind and with two very young children. Despite this, with a lot of help from her mother and a 'can do' positive attitude, Dianne went on to study, achieving her doctorate at Deakin University to become the first woman to be part of the Bionic Eye Program in Australia.[67]

So great is our need to cope with sight loss that we may lose sight of others around us. We do have to consider that other people also have needs, confirming perhaps, that in our subjective focus as we struggle and come to terms with vision loss, we think the world revolves around us. Well, let's be blunt, it doesn't! Coping with sight loss requires a balancing of needs, which we call 'assertiveness'. Not to be confused with 'aggression', where you allow your needs to dominate others, or becoming passive, where you allow your needs to be overridden. For example, by being stoic, 'Oh, don't worry dear, I'm alright!' is a typical passive response..

The unstated unwillingness by those around us to offer help could also be based upon a disbelief, non-acceptance, or simply not being told clearly in an assertive way how they, the partner, can help. Marie in Queensland said, 'I told my relatives I had bad vision, but they just sat in the car and I had to find my way into the shop all by myself, it really was stressful. I don't understand what I've got to do to make them offer to help!' An analysis of Marie's issues that emerged from the group discussion was, that, with residual self-pity, she lacked sufficient confidence to be assertive. She had not directly requested the way in which help should be given. As a consequence, family members remained ambivalent, didn't know what to do and she, in turn was too self-conscious to ask her relatives how to assist. The result: further frustration and disappointment.

Nearly all of the people with vision loss I met over a period of fourteen years who managed their lives successfully, said, 'As difficult as it may seem, education of others in explaining not just what you can or can't see, but how you would prefer them to assist, becomes part of a vision impaired person's life.

Numerous cases are reported of partners leaving because they don't know how to cope. In one group session, Jenny reported, 'When my partner found I had macular degeneration, he couldn't cope with this, that I was like a recently purchased product, in some way defective. I asked him to get out, he did and I was left with two teenage children!' Jenny's husband's attitude is not dissimilar to the treatment described in a book called The Barefoot Surgeon,[68] where people with blindness in Nepal, a third world country, are left to fend for themselves.

In a relationship where a wife refused to make allowances for her vision impaired partner, the man said, 'My partner insists on walking so fast that I can't keep up and she doesn't tell me if steps are coming up. I just feel that I'm being pushed as she doesn't accept that I've got bad sight and won't slow down. I've tried to tell her about what I cannot see, but she doesn't seem to want to listen.'

The above responses, 'that my partner doesn't understand my vision' or 'doesn't want to listen,' are common place. They are either based on a lack of knowledge by one partner on how to assist, or an inability to articulate needs. However, they emphasise the point previously made, that with vision loss, we have to become 'educators of others.' This stage cannot be easily reached when, after a recent diagnosis that says 'you are going blind', you are still in shock, denial, or don't know answers to what you need. Help is at hand, though, in the form of Orientation and Mobility specialists, or simulation glasses.

In one discussion group, a woman was complaining, 'I really think our relationship is finished, I don't get any help from my husband!' She gained tremendous success by using simulation glasses, which mimicked her eye condition. 'I asked him to put them on and go down the back steps. On putting them on he said,

"I can't, I'm too scared to do it!" But after this he was really great and things have changed for the better!'

Sometimes it is just a matter of confidence. In a support group, Mary said that now she had 'become blind,' her plans to travel around Australia with her husband in a caravan were cancelled. The caravan was to be sold. However, after several sessions of peer group therapy, Mary recognised that enjoyment of travel did not depend on sight, and she advised the group that she and her husband had not sold the caravan after all and were going on their 'trip of a lifetime'.

Likewise, Adrian reported that he was losing his sight and felt that he and his partner could no longer go camping as 'I had always done the driving'. He went on to say that 'I felt I couldn't discuss my vision loss with her. But, thanks to hearing what others do, now the wife quite happily drives and it was a matter of realising pride doesn't matter, roles can change!'

Many totally blind people travel overseas independently, go on cruises and enjoy life's experiences, and there are many support services which help. (See Chapter 17, Orientation and Mobility, Dogs versus Canes, Safety and Travel.)

The Response of Friends

There are many mixed messages emerging from friendship stories. While some friends may not know how to handle vision loss and disappear from your life, a group participant said of these aquaintances, 'They become toxic and you are better off without them.' However, others can become closer and more supportive, demonstrating remarkable perception.

There is a well-recognised response if a friend cannot cope: 'Well, It's their problem, not mine!' You might also lose your long-standing friends, but don't see this as caused by your vision loss; it is they who have the acceptance problem. Either they were fair weather friends in the first place, or are fearful, or feel awkward about thinking they might have to assist you and simply don't know how to help.

On the other hand, many people with vision impairment acknowledge that 'best friends have come as a result of blindness'. You can take charge here and train your friends with sighted guide techniques (see Chapter 17, Orientation and Mobility), so that friends too can be confident in going out with you. A peer, the late Justin Simpson from Canberra, with total sight loss said, 'I found that when I explained to my friends how they could help me, they were all supportive. They had no hesitation in taking me to the toilet or ordering drinks when it was my turn to buy!' This view was supported by a woman with retinal dystrophy in Queensland, who said that, 'After realising I could tell my friends that I had bad eyesight, they look after me, help me with the stairs of my club and get meals, drinks and everything!'

Quite logically, if you are angry, bitter and twisted, no one wishes to befriend you, but if you are friendly and happy, others will feel comfortable with your company. Remember the old maxim: Cry and we cry alone, laugh and the world laughs with you.

Often uncertainty of how to help is highlighted when friends are sharing photographs of their children or holidays and passing them around for comment. 'I was so upset because I couldn't see the photos,' said one woman with macular degeneration, 'that I just went into my room and cried!' In so doing she indicated she had not yet come to terms with her sight loss, and illustrated the awkwardness we might experience when still unsure of what to say or how to react.

On the other hand, sighted people may also become embarrassed about handing pictures around or going to the movies. I've often heard friends say, 'There's no point in going to the movies if you can't see them!' However, once Audio Description (AD) is explained and you can use a Companion Card for them to gain free entry, this view changes. Some friends apologise, 'I'm sorry, I forgot you can't see!' Or 'I shouldn't ask if you read books!' These are typical sighted people's perspectives when they do not know how a vision impaired person actually functions.

It's quite common for a sighted person to say something like, 'I realise you can't see my photos anymore!' and then feel embarrassed because of the awkwardness of the situation. If someone passes you photos, don't pretend, take the initiative and say openly, for example, 'I'm sorry, my eyesight is so bad now that I cannot see details anymore. Would you mind describing the photo to me? I'd really love to catch up!' The person who is so proud of her or his offspring or recent trip will invariably take time to explain, and the person with vision impairment, can still participate.

Family communication can be managed by:

- using clear, open and honest communication
- explaining in clear and simple terms what you see and don't see. If you meet with disbelief, you may have to do this several times, or use simulation glasses

- developing assertiveness skills in asking for help and saying clearly what kind of help you need. This may depend upon you knowing what works best, and the experience of other vision impaired people or specialist staff may need to be accessed to provide this information
- helping others to understand the difference between total blindness and various degrees of low vision, by using Simulation glasses or getting support from an Orientation and Mobility Specialist
- explaining the audio and technology you use which enables you to participate. Take advantage of the Companion Card to ask friends to go with you to events
- understanding a family member maybe also be grieving and need support. Your family may need time to accept and adjust to changes.

(6)

Things that Disempower Us

'When you give yourself permission to communicate what matters to you in every situation you will have peace despite rejection or disapproval. Putting a voice to your soul helps you to let go of the negative energy of fear and regret'.

Shannon L. Alder, author

'Emotional hurt is the price a person has to pay in order to be independent.'
Haruki Murakami, What I Talk About When I Talk About
Running

Asking for Help

Even many people with no disability find asking for help difficult. There are many reasons for this and include, not wanting to disturb another, feeling embarrassed, feeling inadequate, or that you should be able to do it independantly. When vision loss makes asking others to assist imperative, for many people this task becomes a major challenge. Yet, on a positive note, it has been my own experience that asking the public generally to help me in Australia and overseas has been uplifting! Like many others with vision impairment, I have found strangers are only too willing to assist, particularly when you can, in a friendly way, provide — with a smile — a clear request for what help you need.

I can recall many instances of such help, but one in particular stands out. I was in Italy in 1999, the train was late, there was no information desk in the station and I had missed my transfer bus, last one for the day. It was raining torrentially from a late summer storm, it was nearly dark, the nearest hotel was over 500 metres away across a park now fading into darkness and I had no umbrella. I was stressed and, to say the least, things looked pretty grim. In desperation I approached a young girl in the reasonable belief she had learned English at school and asked if she spoke English. She did and upon explaining my predicament, she promptly organised for a taxi, a travelling companion to share the ride and turned what could have been disaster, into success. Thank you to that girl and all those unknown people who help. I achieve my goals because of you!

Let's face it, people who are blind or vision impaired depend heavily upon support of others. Obtaining support when you need it is one of the key skills required to maintain independence.

Asking for help is one of our greatest initial challenges because it implies lack of capacity, or weakness. However, the sooner we get over this apprehension, the sooner we are on a pathway to success. Nevertheless, it is incumbent upon us to acknowledge with appreciation any offer of help, even if not required, and avoid being rude. Recently, callers to a radio station complained of how when offering to assist a blind man, they were told to 'F ... off!' Okay, so the blind person was angry, perhaps anti-social, but people are not obliged to assist and maybe next time they won't offer when it might be really needed.

On a broader level, our Australian and other International communities depend upon a very large pool of Volunteers. In Australia over six million volunteers create an economic value of an estimated $A260 billion.[69] So, people with sight loss are not alone in needing help.

Asking for help can also be particularly difficult for those who have been carers and supporters of a family, or have held a high-profile position in the work force. They are usually the person who provides help for others, and it can be hard to change roles.

Even for the average person asking others for help isn't easy, although with their acknowledged social skills, women are recognised to be better at sharing problems than men.[70]

On the surface, it appears contradictory to say that in asking others to help, you are actually increasing your independence. As Peer Justin Simpson, from Canberra said, 'Independence is the capacity to have choice. That is you either can ask for help or not. However, if you do not accept that others can assist, you are not allowing yourself to have that choice.'

If we think about it for a minute, our lives are not totally independent anyway. We are not Robinson Crusoe living alone upon an island and, in any event, in his case, Man Friday came along and gave a helping hand. We live in a world of interdependence, relying upon a community of services and supports. In a typical example provided by group participants, we wrongly believe independence means being able to drive a car and go shopping, yet all facets depend upon a hierarchy of community services. However, giving up driving in a car-dependent community is difficult and remains a major disruptive force and stressor when vision loss occurs.

Factors preventing us from asking for help include:

- pride, self-pity and feeling ashamed or embarrassed
- a fear of losing independence
- not knowing what to ask
- lack of knowledge about what to ask for
- possible role changes
- shyness, or undue politeness, feeling a burden, in asking strangers
- being judged as disabled or uninformed.

It's remarkable to think that when our modern supermarkets were designed, one of the most important considerations was that, following results of surveys, people said they did not like asking a grocer about products and their properties, because this displayed a consumer's lack of knowledge. It was discovered that capable shoppers thought they should already know the answers, and asking for advice from the shopkeeper suggested they lacked a perceived practical capacity. So the problem of asking for help is not new, perhaps universal and not just confined to those with vision impairment. We may also hold concerns that others are too busy to help and our needs are not so important. Ah! Here comes the stoic again.

In coming to terms with the need to ask for help, it is also important to remember, that usually, if someone else had asked you to assist, you would be only too glad to assist and feel pleased for having done so. That's how most people will react to you and it is now your turn to receive some help — and that's okay!

Once you have accepted that asking others for assistance actually offers independence and confidence, this will assist you in allowing situations that previously may have embarrassed you, to diminish and be less important. Actually, vision impaired people who are relaxed within themselves will say, 'It doesn't matter what others say, or think!' But then they have crossed the stormy passage, completed their Odyssey and feel comfortable within their skin. They understand what disempowerment means and have learned to be assertive.

While finding out what help is out there enhances our options for living, the way others respond, including the words they use, can make us feel put down, an unintentional inferior/superior relationship. We need to understand this relationship to become assertive. (See Reflective or Active Listening) But even using assertive behaviour, sometimes really silly things happen.

Some Examples of Sheer Nincompoopery

Despite the tension encountered when facing strangers, yes, we need to laugh. As sad as it might appear, there are sheer acts of what is best called nincompoopery committed when sighted people, confronted by those with vision loss, don't know what to do or say, or they should know better, or when people with vision impairment think they can do it all themselves. There are many examples of sighted people just taking over. For instance, John in regional Victoria reported, 'I was just standing on the footpath waiting for my friend when a complete stranger came up, grabbed my arm and said, "Let me take you across the road", and before I could think, there I was and I didn't even have the chance to say stop. There I was left there, on the wrong side!' Silly isn't it? But this sort of thing happens more often than you'd like to think. When waiting for a tram, I am often asked if I want to cross the road. Why? Isn't the tram stop obvious? But, there's no point displaying exasperation, or sarcasm. Yes, people are being kind and we must thank them and value this spirit.

Yet, it keeps on rolling on! In a recent telephone dog handlers' discussion group,[71] a participant texted

'I am so glad Sadie [a dog guide] and I were able to provide such high value entertainment this Saturday afternoon on the grass at Sydney Central Station while Sadie engaged in the simple art of crapping in a bag. Before I knew it, this crowd gathers around us. A man is explaining at the top of his voice about what a genius invention this toilet harness is and there are phones out pointing towards us ... I'm like, Give the girl some privacy guys!' Then to cap it all off, 'This trumped up security guard came barrelling over to me and said I just had a report your dog took a shit on my lawn! To which I replied, yep right here in this bag, handing it to him!'

Another participant said this happens to them too, and her dog guide, Ilka, gets 'performance anxiety'! However, some humorous reactions from others in the group included the comment, 'Charge tickets next time!' and 'Should have opened up your suitcase to welcome donations!'

In further examples of sighted people just not 'getting it', Amanda who worked for a Blind Sports organisation supporting walking groups and organising tours for people who are blind or vision impaired, said that in making reservations with a motel for a bus tour, the reception lady said when finding out the tourists were vision impaired, 'Oh, some rooms won't be suitable as they have stairs leading up to them!' Really! People who are blind and vision impaired can't walk up or down stairs? Remember Mike Hingson and his dog Roselle walking down 78 flights unaided? But, it gets worse. In talking to a coordinator for other disability community support groups, Amanda was shocked to hear her say, 'We don't have those [blind] people on these walks. We have had those people before! If you like them that much, you take them yourself!'

Then there's the case of a totally blind young man in regional Victoria in the books of an employment agency, being offered the role of — yes, can you believe it — as a driver for a pizza delivery van! Sadly, at age thirty-three, he still couldn't find work yet he has excellent communication skills. We really have to question the role of disability employment agencies when these outcomes occur.

For most sighted onlookers, vision loss is not visible and this creates disbelief or incredulity. People say, 'You don't look blind, or act blind!' Or 'Your eyes don't look blind!' Which logically raises the question, what is 'being blind' supposed to look like?' Raylene in Queensland advised, 'A teller in my bank said, "Your eyes look normal!"' Comments similar to this appear to be part of the essential confusion people with sight hold about blindness. Unless there is actual physical damage, or where the eyes don't focus, for the vast majority of people with vision impairment eyes look normal.

One of the most annoying conversation openers is, 'I bet you don't recognise my voice.' All blind people deal with variations of this opener. Some friends of mine — yes, they still are! — like to trick me by remaining silent to see if I recognise them. They cop a sharp tongue when this happens. It takes a good deal of self-confidence to respond, 'No, I'm sorry, I do not!' and then stop speaking while continuing to look at the person. I have often wanted to retort, 'No, but if you were someone important I would!'

We Do Have to Laugh

As well as tears and tales of heartbreak, my discussion groups were also moments of spontaneous humour, which always provided relief and real joy. Here are some anecdotes that prove being blind has its lighter side. And yes, they are true!

A woman with very, very poor sight, was seen in a main street of Melbourne, attempting to post a letter into a woman wearing a bright pillar box red overcoat.

A woman with a new dog guide and unfamiliar with her hound, began to wonder why it took so long to get down to her local shopping centre until she realised the dog was just going around and around a street roundabout.

Maurice Gleeson, totally blind from early youth with retinal detachment, now President of Blind Sports and Recreation Victoria, tells how one day he was caught in a rush hour crowd at a train station. 'A girl in a hurry just crashed straight into me and in exasperation cried out, "Oh, Jesus Christ!" To which I said, "I'm terribly sorry to disappoint you, but I'm afraid I can't help you!''' Humour so often, comes to the rescue.

But, it is not all one-way. People with vision impairment contribute to misunderstanding by remaining in denial and not using ID badges or a white cane. Yes, they don't have to, but Susan in Melbourne who had very poor vision thought she could manage to find herself a seat on a suburban train. She peered into a carriage of her train at Flinders Street station, and thought it was completely empty. 'So in I marched, took a seat and yes, can you believe it? I sat on the lap of the only man, yes, the only man, seated in the carriage! Oh, did I think I was a fool!'

In another instance, Jan from Victoria, too embarrassed to use a white cane, or ask for help, was one evening on her way to rest rooms in a hotel where a corridor was lined with mirrors. 'I kept stepping aside and apologising to a stranger, only to eventually realise it was me reflected in the mirror that I was apologising to!' Jan's not alone, I have done the same when walking into a mirrored entrance hall to a function, walked up hand outstretched, to introduce myself!

Until vision loss becomes pronounced, there is actually no requirement for disclosure. This, combined with the fact that the vast majority of those with a vision disability are not totally blind, confuses the sighted and adds to their discombobulation. In talking about a boat trip on the Gippsland Lakes, Brenda, who has macular degeneration, relayed the following, 'As we were about to disembark the ferry, my husband took me by the arm and led me to the ship's rails. I overheard someone gasp, then another said, "Oh, Is it safe? Can she swim?" Exasperated with this nonsense, my husband turned and said, "It's OK, she usually jumps overboard and swims to shore!"'

Dealing with Disempowering Situations

If we accept that there are really two worlds, one of the sighted and one for the vision impaired, how then might we bring the two together?

First, to recognise that all people who say they are 'blind' or 'can't see', are not black blind. That people using a white cane are not necessarily totally blind. That vision impairment means difficulty seeing, or that partial sight which may inhibit normal responses doesn't mean total blindness, or that you are stupid. That people with vision loss might be slower, peer at signs, appear lost or disorientated, but this doesn't mean they are dumb, or lacking capacity.

Second, that people with vision impairment are required to be educators as well as be assertive — that is, to be quite determined to insist that they get levels of service they need, but be prepared to explain why and how assistance is to be provided. For example, like asking to hold a person's elbow with Sighted Guide techniques. This is part of the requirement when becoming vision impaired, to become an educator. A recent example illustrates this point. A man made a telephone inquiry to a service provider and told the customer service officer that he was calling because he could not access the internet, that he had poor vision and that he had lost his customer card. 'Okay,' was the response, 'I understand, I'll send you a form in the mail to fill in and send back!' This response, of course, was completely unhelpful but typical of a normal sighted world. It took perseverance to make the point, 'Sending a form is of no use, I can't fill it in.' Finally the customer service officer got the message and agreed to fill in the application himself, confirming personal details with the client. It is therefore important that people with vision impairment be assertive and request this level of support when needed. Increasing use of the Internet and requests that sales orders, or application forms be filled in on line, also disempower people with vision loss. However, re-skilling and training can mostly overcome this.

In many cases people just don't listen, and patience and assertiveness are required. A typical response of the sighted customer service operator is, having just been told the customer is blind, 'You will have to identify yourself, bring in your driver's licence.' Person with vision impairment, 'I don't have a drivers licence.' .

In Britain recently, an example of misunderstanding — well, let's call it for what it really was, prejudice — occurred when a sighted person uploaded a photo to Facebook of a lady holding a white cane while also using their smartphone. It had the caption, 'If you can see what's wrong say I see it!' Suggesting this person was faking blindness. How could someone who is blind also use a phone? This extraordinary assumption was surely based on ignorance. But three further people with vision impairment rang the BBC to report that they also had similar experiences, accusing people with vision impairment of faking it. By March 2019, this photo had been shared more than 33,000 times.[72]

What is plainly misunderstood by the above observers and others, is that assistive technology and text to speech audio features such as 'Voice Over' in iPhone and 'Talk Back' in Androids, plus many other accessible audio apps, have made this technology completely accessible and essential for people with vision loss. They don't have to see it to use it, and it's life-changing!

What is not so funny, is that medical professionals don't always respond effectively either. Clients frequently reported being told, 'Well you are going blind, get over it!' That was the rather brutal comment from one doctor following diagnosis. Paul from Victoria told how his doctor asked, 'Have you got your driver's licence?' When he unsuspectingly handed it over, the doctor just tore it up in front of him and his partner. 'There was no discussion of what to do next,' Paul said, 'or even how I was to travel 200K home to the country.'

My doctor simply said, 'I can't do any more for you!' and left me, eyes blurred from eyedrops, to go home with no referral to further support. This experience is not uncommon. Helen from New South Wales told of this form of dismissal when she said of her experience, 'I saw two ophthalmologists. The first just smiled and said I had RP and could no longer drive and offered no other explanation! And the other said I would not be able to drive before long, but also offered no information or advice on where to go or where to get support. I was devastated!' You really have to wonder why the medical practitioner doesn't explain what is happening.

Jenny was born with low vision and just accepted this as her life. She was only told at age 31 by an optometrist working with the Royal Victorian Institute for the Blind (RVIB) that she was 'Legally Blind' and had been so 'from early childhood'! This designation would have allowed her access to government benefits. An ophthalmologist I saw when I was younger didn't even tell my parents, which would have been so helpful to them and in my case, that I would have been eligible for government pension and other supports for the past 15 years!' explained Jenny.

Some doctors simply lack communication skills (The bedside manner,) in conveying bad news to their patients. In any event, just leaving patients to their own ends is simply unprofessional. It does seem inexplicable why in these cases information about the patient's health was not conveyed appropriately. If you feel your doctor does not communicate well, or you are left doubting in any way, always seek a second opinion. Ask your friends who they see, or ask your vision impaired service agency who to go to.

Words that Disempower Us

A common statement made by participants in my discussion groups was that sighted people say things that are insensitive. Some examples are:

'Why don't you go into a home?'

'You should use a white cane!'

'Why don't you get a guide dog?'

'Why don't you get new glasses?'

Many of these statements are made with good intent, of concern, looking after your interests, being interested. But they are actually put-downs. Such inquiries place one person in a superior position to the other.

We ourselves may respond to others in a similar vein in other circumstances. for example, in talking to someone who is ill, how often might we say, 'Have you tried a certain medication?' Or 'Why don't you go to Doctor Bloggs?' Or 'Try using this medication.' We typically say these things as everyday responses without thinking about their effect. We are just trying to be helpful.

Word such as, 'You should', 'You must', 'Why don't you?' Or just 'Why?) unwittingly place the inquisitor in a superior position to the other by requesting an answer. It might be an answer we don't want to provide, or don't know what to say and feel uncomfortable in being expected to respond.

Frequently out of politeness, or not being sure what to say, or perhaps unaware of the impact of what they are saying, friends as well as strangers use comparisons or platitudes. For example, 'I know exactly how you feel!' Or 'I know what it's like, I have worn glasses all my life" Or 'I'm blind without my glasses!' might be genuine, but are of no value to people with serious vision loss. Others attempt to place themselves in a sympathetic position by using comparative statements such as, 'Oh, you're lucky you do not have cancer' (or Alzheimer's etc), as they attempt to console. Other banalities are based on the supposition people with blindness have developed superior skills; 'You must have amazing hearing!' Or 'An amazing memory!' are frequently heard.

People attempt to hide their discomfort by claiming there must be advantages in losing sight, for instance, 'You must be so brave, I really admire you!' Or 'You are amazing!' Or 'I don't know how you can do it!' can be annoying when a person with vision loss is just getting on with life. But, a sighted person cannot imagine how they could do it if blind.

Other typical responses suggesting ignorance when dealing with differences include running off to fetch a person with vision impairment a wheelchair, or offering a seat without asking whether you might prefer one. Sometimes diminutives such as 'dear' or 'love,' or 'darl' are used as part of a parochial idiom; but these can be quite patronising. The best rule for people with sight is to remember that people with vision loss are just like you. Ask yourself, how would I like to be spoken to?

But all of the above is what many participants of my discussion groups and I have to deal with once we mention having a vision impairment. Understanding how we normally respond to each other in everyday conversations is important if we are to withstand the negative, sometimes hurtful, impacts. For many, the solution lies in changing the way we typically respond when listening.

Reflective or Active Listening

Listening to others in an empathic way is called active or reflective listening. When you listen in this way, you do not express a view on what you think a person should do, but give choice and empowerment to the other. Much peer training is based on this idea, where it is better to give your experience on how you solved a similar issue, than tell a person what they should do.

When we listen to someone, we respond in different ways depending on the situation and personalities involved. As identified by Dr David W. Johnson, the five main ways are:

1. judgemental/evaluative/advice — directive
2. interpretive/explanatory — teaching
3. supportive/soothing/reassuring — sympathetic
4. probing/questioning/information seeking — inquisitive
5. understanding — empathic.

The least used response is, you guessed it! Number 5! Empathy means simply that we stand in the shoes of another. Dr Johnson says, 'That our life's experiences have given us understanding, which means you do not say, 'I understand how difficult it must be!', when you actually do not.

What is interesting is that the first four of the above responses place us in a superior position to the other and allow us not to engage intimately with the recipient. Most change is achieved when both conversationalists are on an equal footing, on a personal level as human beings. You don't have to have an answer — just being there, offering understanding is helpful and empowering. Remember what it is like to have only one good friend who listens. Reflective listening is much more than just hearing. It involves, decoding, interpreting and understanding the meaning and significance of the experience.'[73]

Day-to-day Matters that Disempower People with Vision Loss

Apart from our communications with each other, some day-to-day disempowering situations for people with vision impairment include:

- giving up driving
- not being able to read
- not identifying faces
- losing choice
- not accessing information
- giving up work
- involuntary role changes
- physical barriers
- using public transport for the first time
- a disbelief by others that you are vision impaired
- being criticised as 'too stubborn'
- being told what to do

- decisions made about your future without you being involved — 'You should go into an aged care home!'

How Can Sighted People Help?

If you are sighted, there is absolutely nothing wrong in approaching and asking a person with vision impairment if they need help, although keep in mind that although they might appear lost, slow or confused, they may not actually be so. They might be thinking or just needing to take things slowly, but it is still better to ask than walk on, not sure of what to say.

Responding is quite simple. To ask, 'Do you need some help?' or 'May I help you?' will allow the person with vision loss to accept or reject this initial offer. Don't worry or be offended if they say 'No'. If they say 'Yes', then simply asking 'How can I assist?' leaves it open for the person with sight loss to invite assistance.

In a social setting, it is acceptable to ask a vision impaired person, 'Do you have total sight loss?' Or 'Can you see a little?' Then, 'Do you need any assistance?' Or 'May I assist you?' can naturally follow.

Keep your inquiry honest and simple. It is best not to inquire, 'What's wrong, or what eyesight condition do you have?' This becomes quite intrusive, but also opens up the opportunity for the pedantic to offer too much boring detail. You might already be aware of the preparedness of others to neurotically talk about their illnesses. For further details on how to assist people who are blind or vision impaired, see Chapter 17, Orientation and Mobility.

From the perspective of onlookers, friends and family members responding to disability, ask: 'You sound upset, annoyed, aggravated.' etc. Or 'You look ... Tired, hurt, upset, etc. Tell me more ...'

The object is to encourage the person to identify what is upsetting them and whether they can control it and you can actually assist.

In conclusion, work with people with vision impairment and seek solutions together. Don't just assume something or take over. Rather than assuming you know the answer, you simply need to listen.

7

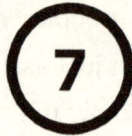

The Psychology of Blindness and Trauma Impact

'The deeper we go in the search for who I am, the deepest truth is that part of what I do, my work, hobbies, family, beliefs, or even my gender ... is not who I am ... it is my relationship to other people ... it is indivisible. In the search for who I am, the essential truth, the magic moment for all of us in the search for who I am, is that I am part of you, we are all part of each other, a species indivisible.'

Hugh Mackay, psychologist

'Life is ten percent what you experience and ninety percent how you respond to it.'
Dr Dorothy M. Neddermeyer, Author, educator in health and wellness.

Why Discuss Trauma?

Clients often came to a group session saying, 'I went to a psychologist and they weren't any help. They didn't understand what vision loss is like!' This was how clients saw it, the ongoing nature of grief which accompanies sight loss, a loss as powerful as that experienced by people losing a loved one, but not diminishing, as they have to live with it on a daily basis, not as the onlooker, but as the subject of a 'living death'.

Many people experiencing gradual loss of sight, when talking about how they felt, were also surprised to hear their feelings were similar to those usually experienced after a sudden traumatic event. Their frustrations, anxieties, anger, feelings of bitterness, resentment and bewilderment, their sense that life had let them down, were commonplace. For these reasons, I think it's helpful to discuss what constitutes trauma and what psychologists say about it.

Trauma does not have to be connected with dramatic events such as accidents, war, fires, floods or other disasters. The announcement by a doctor that you have an incurable eye disease is a deeply distressing or disturbing experience involving life changes for which you are ill-prepared, and trauma can result.

While we await a cure, or remain hoping for some magical therapy, we may be reluctant to accept there is another way of doing things and therefore remain in what psychologist Elisabeth Kübler-Ross called, a grief/trauma curve. The grief and trauma of losing partial sight was expressed when clients in discussion groups said:

'I thought my life was over.'

'I felt I was halfway across a river and couldn't move forward or back!'

'There's no point in living now I can't see my family!'

Feelings of sorrow, grief and loss apply to everyone of course and are not confined to vision loss. However, the majority of people I encountered who underwent sudden sight loss, or lost their sight later in life, spoke about their experience as one of intense trauma. Mohammed from Victoria, in his mid-forties, experienced instant and total sight loss as a result of detached retinas in both eyes. He described the devastating impact as, 'It was like falling into a deep black sea at midnight and drowning!'

When the opportunity arose for clients to talk about these feelings and hear others talking similarly, group participants invariably expressed profound relief. The simple process of sharing emotions with others normalised things. Typical emotions identified were:

- anger, a state of shock which can prevent taking action, or alternatively spur action — I won't put up with this!
- feelings of resentment and frustration leading to inertia and anxiety — 'It's all too difficult!'
- bewilderment, sadness, regrets and depression — 'I would prefer to die!', 'I wish there was a cure!'
- fear, a warning as well as a motivator for action — 'I'm afraid to go out!'
- hurt, loss of self-esteem, blame and lack of confidence — 'I'm useless, I'm not as good as I used to be!'

- denial and avoidance — 'There's someone worse off than me!'

Often it is the stoic expectation that 'I must keep on', or that 'my vision loss is not as bad as someone else,' or 'I must not give up,' etc, contribute to a suppression of deeper emotions. Being able to talk about these feelings is, as many of my group participants said, life changing!

Other typical responses include:

- I am used to doing things without having to ask for help; asking makes me feel useless or ineffectual.
- Having to deal with strangers when I ask for assistance makes me feel vulnerable.
- I am naturally shy, and I'm challenged by the idea of having to be assertive when asking for help from strangers.
- Hurt and grief make me feel I want to crawl into a hole and hope the world will go away.
- I've found that professionals on whom I rely are unhelpful, intolerant or even patronising, which makes me feel even more disillusioned and disempowered than I was before.
- I feel cut off from friends and have lost interest in activities.
- I have trouble sleeping, even though I feel exhausted.

The consensus view of psychologists supports the opinion that it is better for our health and wellbeing that we open up and express feelings of grief, to bring these emotions out in the open rather than keeping them contained. In this context, I found that women are better prepared to discuss emotional issues and more likely to attend a discussion group than men.[74] Women are five times more likely to cry than men,[75] and men more likely to hide or disguise their emotional stress as a 'weakness'. (See Chapter 13, Teenagers, Men, Issues of Vision Loss and Socialisation.)

Other negative or destructive responses identified in my group sessions included staying busy, bottling things up, using distractions, smoking and drinking alcohol more than usual, and trying to avoid facing their situation. Also expressed were fears about loss of competence, losing capacity for work, hobbies and relationships, with further comments such as, 'Who would want to love a blind man?' (See Chapters 5 and 13.)

Positive Psychology

If, as I have discussed in Chapter 1 and above, in dealing with loss, grief and fears, people are not 'depressed', but through lack of hope for a cure or of reclaiming their former lives, they are experiencing 'Adjustment Disorder'; they are losing focus on the positive — concepts also relevant for mindfulness. (See Chapter 8, Dealing with Worry, Anxiety and Stress.)

With feelings of hopelessness and perhaps learned helplessness, the philosophy of positive psychology becomes applicable.[76] positive psychology is understood to be a 'scientific approach to studying human thoughts, feelings, and behaviour, with a focus on strengths instead of weaknesses, building the good in life instead of repairing the bad, and taking the lives of average people up to great, instead of focusing solely on moving those who are struggling up to "normal"'.[77]

In essence, positive psychology embraces:

1. Positive experiences (like happiness, joy, inspiration and love).

2. Positive states and traits (like gratitude, resilience and compassion).

3. Applying positive principles to whole organisations.

Why then is this relevant to vision loss? As a field of practice, positive psychology spends much of its time thinking about topics highly relevant to sight loss, like character strengths, optimism, life satisfaction, happiness, wellbeing, gratitude, compassion (as well as self-compassion), self-esteem and self-confidence, hope, and elevation. Many, if not most of these feelings are experienced when vision loss occurs. These topics are studied in order to learn how to help people flourish and live their best lives, issues directly relevant to loss of vision. The understanding we can carry on doing things differently to how we did so before doesn't diminish the person.

A proponent of this philosophy, Professor Lea Asher, says, 'we need to consider concepts of grace, of being gracious. Of owning up to errors and mistakes and not hiding them. To learn how to disengage. In confronting things which come your way, don't be reactive — be proactive'. That in dealing with stress, 'Acknowledge the little things in your life where you are successful. Ask, what have I done successfully?'[78]

However, to respond positively, as Professor Asher says, is very hard when we feel isolated, embarrassed, shameful or hurt by a disability which we didn't ask for, and we don't know where to go or how to keep on going. We may not be able to understand or easily explain our loss, especially when genetics and family dynamics are involved, but as the chapters in this book illustrate, by re-skilling, adopting technology and accepting difference, a full and rewarding life can be regained. One example of how little it actually took to re-direct focus and feelings of positivity, was when I rang clients. In most cases they had Mobile phone numbers. I always asked, 'What type of phone have you got?' If the client said a Smart phone, I'd then ask, 'Do you use or know about SIRI, or Voice Over?' if it was an Iphone. If they didn't I'd explain it, or email instructions with amazing results. People thinking themselves shut out, suddenly realized they could now use their phone, read documents texts and search the Internet, their world was accessible again.

Disappointment, Pity and other Responses

The struggle to 'beat it, or fight it', or the self-doubt or self-consciousness which comes in admitting you are not feeling well or energised, or admitting that you have a disability, may mean we remain in a state of avoidance of our basic emotions where we cannot express them and thus, in this state, remain traumatised. This was the situation I commonly found with clients in my group discussions.

The above responses are not confined to loss of sight, of course. As Beyond Blue states on its website (www.beyond blue. org.au or phone 1300 22 46 36), emotional responses of trauma can include, 'Shock, disbelief, sadness, distress, shame, blame, numbness, anxiety, guilt, fear, regret, anger, helplessness, suicidal'. The overwhelming nature of anxiety can cause us to question life and its meaning.

A common feeling associated with giving up seeing others and the non-fulfilment of expectations such as work, hobbies or seeing your family grow up, was expressed as disappointment. 'I was so disappointed not to see the film, read that book, see my grandchild etc.' It is a softer term often used to cover deeper feelings of sadness. In dealing with this disappointment associated with loss, psychologist Eve Waters[79] notes that 'we may not know how to stop dwelling on issues', to 'distract ourselves' and ask, 'What can I now do to take my mind off the issue?' That in a state of shock we may not think of even simple things to do which distract us, like sport, reading with audio books, walking with a companion, going out with friends, and so on.

Conversely, others around us as noted above, in trying to help, may express pity, rather than empathy, and make us react defensively. If you become aware of this, you have choices to make as previously mentioned, for example:

- Avoid negative friends, unless they have already avoided you.
- Develop assertiveness skills by asking others to assist you in the way you require, not in a way they assume is correct.
- Adopt an educator's approach, this needs patience.
- Re-skill yourself to regain confidence, this takes time.

What Psychologists Say

In commenting on the impact of trauma, psychologist Anne Leadbeater, noted that 'Intense trauma and hope can co-exist together. The main concern is when people do not express their grief but remain silent!'[80] Adding to this understanding, trauma expert, Clinical Psychologist, Dr. Rob Gordon[81] also notes that 'Traumatic incidents may trigger different emotional, physical and psychological reactions. The way you recover from trauma depends on many things, such as the type and severity of the traumatic event, how much support is available, other stressors in your life, your level of resilience, and whether you have experienced traumatic experiences before'.

A large component of grief counselling is based upon bereavement. Current thinking in psychology now believes that the six stages of grief proposed in earlier years by Elisabeth Kübler-Ross were followed too literally and seen as sequential stages. I agree with this conclusion, as I found that with vision loss, the changing nature and complexity of poor vision, regular setbacks and associated feelings, varied over time, location and with the individual. As a client progressed, perhaps taking on greater challenges, there was a need to revisit emotional stages.

In a recent example of how psychologists now consider grief with loss of a loved one, Clinical Psychologist, Dr William Worden suggests that grieving should be considered as an 'active process that involves engagement with four tasks and seven other considerations'.[82] Taking into account and acknowledging Dr Worden's principles, I set out these factors and include further considerations which accommodate the vision loss experience:

A. 'Acceptance might come in stages,' boosted by recognising success in undertaking daily tasks differently to how they were carried out before. While Professor Christopher Hall Maps states that 'most people ultimately adapt well to bereavement,' sight loss because it is brought home every waking hour, every day, possibly deteriorating and relentless, may inhibit this recovery. It is as if death has occurred within a person, but no funeral or ceremony has taken place to provide an end point. As a result, grief becomes internalised. Outsiders can also look on not knowing what to do or say, or even grow tired of listening to the person with vision impairment complaining of how difficult things are. At the same time, in attempting to keep going and maintain social and societal expectations, an individual's resources are challenged.

B. 'Processing the hurt accompanying grief,' will depend upon age, personality, family supports and character and degree of vision loss. It will be a process of going through it to get to the other side not avoiding it. This may involve feelings of exhaustion, loss of sleep, appetite, focus and making decisions (See Chapter 9 on health issues.) Taking good personal care and being kind to yourself are important. Avoid 'toxic friends' and use distractors such as exercise, music, study, friendships and social outlets.

C. 'In adjusting,' to a world without sight, or with restricted sight including both internal, external and spiritual adjustments, Is where re-skilling, mobility, tasks and technology and use of audio devices (books and newspapers) becomes so important in creating a belief in yourself. This re-skilling doesn't necessarily stop but a base level of skills can offer confidence and capacity to remain independent in the home, or community (See Chapters 16 & 17.). The shock of sight loss can also affect our capacity for acceptance. Concepts of unfairness blame or self-pity, can occur to slow down or even prevent acceptance.

D. 'Regaining a former life,' of work, family and other interests as you create a new life, does not mean rejection of the former life. What I call, 'being comfortable with yourself, comfortable within your skin, that blindness or vision loss are not a fate worse than death!' is the understanding of acceptance.

Worden's seven determining factors which require consideration include:

(1) who you, the previous person, was as an individual; (2) the nature of attachments to family, work, friends etc; (3) how sight loss occurred i.e. sudden or gradual, accident or genetic; (4) historical i.e. prior family experiences with sight loss or genetic influences; (5) personality and culture variables; (6) social mediators, the likelihood that former friends may dessert you and the need and confidence to ask others for help; and (7) concurrent stressors.

Dealing with Partial Vision Loss

I often describe having partial vision as being in a 'limbo land', neither sighted nor blind, living in a foggy neutral world of grey blurredness, of being and feeling neither here nor there, losing touch with one's original identity. In many instances, remaining sight may slowly diminish and vary from day to day. Seemingly okay one day, then worse the next. In such circumstances, grief and regrets do not go away with a flick of a switch, or the blink of an eye. Typical responses reported by clients with partial sight include:

'Just when I think my eyes are stable, they seem to get worse and I can't see what I could yesterday!'

'All I see is a blur, I just don't want to get out of bed.'

'What's the point of trying to pretend I'm happy when I'm not.'

'Every morning I wake up and realise that my eyes haven't changed and my life remains in a fog and I feel my eyes are getting worse!'

From another perspective, frustrated by our diminished sight, we may find we compare ourselves to high 'alpha' achievers, or a world going on without us and this only increases feelings of inadequacy, of being left behind and feeling isolated. As noted in earlier Chapters, high achievers who, although totally blind, or seriously physically impaired, run marathons, climb mountains, skydive, play golf, perform in the paralympics and rise to the top of their profession. It is a natural response to think, 'I couldn't possibly do that!', and this makes us feel more useless than ever. Of course, you don't have to be a high achiever to live a fulfilling life, but noting high achievement does tell us what can be done if we want to.

As acknowledged by many studies, much support comes from families, but when a family itself is in disbelief or denial, this in turn can lead to increased emotional and even physical change in the affected person. However, as psychologist Dr Rob Gordon says, our response to trauma also depends upon the rapidity of onset and our innate capacities to respond. Psychiatrist Dr Colin Murray Parkes states, 'The ideal is to achieve a balance between avoidance and confrontation which enables the person gradually to come to terms with the loss. Until people have gone through the painful process of searching, they cannot "let go" of their attachment ... and move on then review or revise their basic assumptions.'[83]

The reference to 'attachment' (above) is also a major component of the Buddhist philosophy, that becoming too attached to our emotions among other material desires, distorts our mind and thinking, a concept now closely associated with mindfulness. (See Chapter 8, Dealing with Worry, Anxiety and Stress.)

A key for those with vision impairment to bear this burden will naturally depend on how we can adjust, and this in turn depends on factors such as our personality, character, family values, attitudes and knowledge. Qualities such as perseverance and focusing on the present, not the past, come into play.

These qualities are not just relevant for the newly diagnosed. Perseverance is exemplified by Cheryl, a peer from Queensland, who had total vision loss extending over 20 years. She was required to use all positive qualities after relocating to a new single-level home in 2018. Cheryl said, 'Even though the Agent had described my new home, I found it totally disorientating and upsetting, even trying to find main rooms. I had to get an Orientation and Mobility Specialist in to train me within my home and kitchen, how the entrance was located to the bench, how cupboards worked and how rooms led off my main focal point of the kitchen bench. It took several weeks to adjust.'

The belief that we actually can grow, become stronger and more capable as a result of this experience, is an outcome often too far away to believe and accept in the beginning, but, as now frequently stated, life doesn't end with blindness or vision loss.

As discussed in Chapter 6 (Things that Disempower Us), reaching out for solutions becomes very difficult when doctors send patients away with a diagnosis of incurable blindness without referring their patient to further rehabilitation and emotional support services.[84] If any plea can be made, it is for greater enlightenment in this regard. The sooner clients can move to rehabilitation, re-skilling and regaining hope, the less negativity and depression will occur.

Is there a Correct Time to Grieve?

With death, grief for onlookers is intense and, in some instances, deep and lasting. As with Queen Victoria, who, after death of her beloved Albert, spent the remainder of her last forty years in deep mourning, dressed in black. For most of us, there may be ongoing sadness and feelings of loss, but we get on with our lives. We do not get over it, but get through it.

At a funeral, we openly share and express our sadness and grief by hugs, handshakes, stories and tears, then the intense moment of expression is over, but not necessarily gone. It is also important to note that there is no correct time for grief and mourning. It need not be something that we can close the door on and forget about. Grief and mourning and their accompanying emotions — sadness, melancholy, regret, wishful thinking, self-pity, anger and blame, crying, withdrawal and unhappiness, a deep feeling of emotional pain we otherwise can call a broken heart — are all part of normal responses to grief which includes loss of sight. Unrelieved, these feelings can change a character, cause illness, loss of appetite, sleeplessness, affect mental health, roles and relationships, and even change personality. We may withdraw, as things are now just too hard to cope with.

According to psychotherapist Dr Stephanie Dowrick, 'There is no official, or expiry time for grieving. Profound grief is not something we get over. In time we get on, sometimes noting with surprise how much life is still giving to us even while it has been taking so much away. Yet, the truth is that there is no normal way to grieve, nor is there any neat timetable for grief. We step around making no time for the big emotions.'[85]

We may suppress grief in a desire to 'get on with it', but it may resurface at any time or be triggered by an event, sound, smell, picture or rekindled memory. But when we feel it, we need to recognise it and accept that we are emotional beings, and that grief is an important part of normal human emotional make-up.'

Being Different

Being different, or a reluctance to be different, is a normal human characteristic. However, being different as a result of vision loss, is a major issue. However, feeling different, that you are not fitting in, that you must ask for help, use a white cane or ID badge, is also hard for anyone to accept. Being and feeling different because of a disability lies behind the stigma. As Sheila Hockens who had congenital cataracts, said in her autobiography, Emma and I, 'I was, if the truth be known, ashamed of being blind. I refused to use a white stick and hated asking for help! After all, I was a teenage girl and I couldn't bear people to look at me and think I wasn't like them.'

Sheila described all types of disasters, including being too afraid to ask for help in hailing down her bus, then having to walk five miles back to the city centre, describing as 'idiotic' the things that happened, such as running into lamp poles because she couldn't accept that using a cane would help.[86]

As we are creatures of habit and used to social norms, we rely upon body language, how we dress and appearances to know how we and others fit in. This built in reserve, or resistance to change makes us want to fit in rather than be an outsider. Unless we like being regarded as eccentric or Bohemian, or preferring an alternative lifestyle, we mostly don't like being different, and definitely don't like to admit to a perceived difference arising out of disability.

Upon examination, most of the above positions are, of course, superficial, but they do become part of a vision impaired person's thinking. Few are good at recognising and accepting other people upon qualities of their character. As Dr Martin Luther King said in 1963, people 'will not be judged by the color of their skin [or in this case disability] but by the content of their character'.[87]

Facing Change

As Leigh Sales says in her book Any Ordinary Day,[88] 'We have a human bias towards predictability and a sense of certainty comes from believing that things are under control. This is certainly what disappears with unexpected loss.' People feel better about certainty, about knowing what is coming, even if it is painful. It's easier to prepare ourselves when knowing what's in store. Dopamine creates calmness, contentment, feeling comfortable, relieved and sad. Uncertainty feels close to pain and people try to avoid it.'

In facing sheer bewilderment of a different life for which we have received little preparation or training, we may, as a first response, wish it to go away. We may 'hate' it and wish to crawl back into our darkened room, as one client said, 'All I wanted to do was to stay in bed all day with my doona over my head and blinds down to stop the glare!'

Rather than shut yourself away, the better response is to use your fear and anger to motivate yourself to change things As Maribel Steele puts it, 'Being able to express your feelings and let go of pride and being kind to ourselves, are true marks of strength. It will help the beginner to blindness to realise that a lot of what you imagine or might fear is not necessarily going to come true. Your unsettled mind may be trying to retain control, but in second guessing every scenario possible, it is creating even more barriers.'[89]

Often the stigma you feel attached to your personality by others is a perceived stigma: it can't stick to you unless you let it. It truly doesn't matter what others may think. We all want to be happy, and many of us feel unsatisfied with our lives; as Abraham Lincoln said, 'Most people are about as happy as they want to be.' Accordingly, there is no conclusive test for what makes happiness, or that we are all equal in these feelings. Happiness is subjective, but a good grounding for moving on are empowerment models as suggested by psychologists Eve Waters and Professor Lea Asher, and the concepts of Positive Psychology, which in summary are: to focus on positive things, joy, inspiration, love and resilience, not to dwell on problems, to distract yourself from negativity, acknowledge what causes stress, take action, acknowledge simple successes, don't be reactive, be proactive, and choose how you want to be.

In the midst of our struggle to maintain ourselves, we need to remember that those around us may also be suffering loss, grief and shock over what is happening. Families can also be in denial, fearful of an unknown future, witnessing personality and role changes, or fear and blame over genetic causes. Grief is a multi-layered response and affects us all; it is not restricted to disability. It is easy, then, for a 'them and us' attitude to emerge. 'Sighted people don't understand my vision loss!' and 'Sighted people don't get it!' are typical responses from those with vision loss when trying to explain wat they can or can't see.

Another cause of grief stems from our sense of failure, and accompanying blame. That our faulty genes, or our neglect in looking after ourselves (for example, diabetes), or our inability to cope, is our fault. But as Sally Capp, Lord Mayor of Melbourne said, 'Failure is not fatal! We should embrace failure! As the somewhat tired cliché states, 'We learn from our mistakes. To deny them and pretend or hope they don't exist is the failure!'[90]

It is therefore through knowledge — an understanding of what is happening to our vision, health and emotions –which forms the pathway for the empowerment required to move forward again and take up solutions.

(8)

Dealing with Worry, Anxiety and Stress

'Our anxiety does not empty tomorrow of its sorrows, but only empties today of its strengths.'

C. H. Spurgeon, pastor and author

'Anxiety's like a rocking chair. It gives you something to do, but it doesn't get you very far.'

Jodi Picoult, Sing You Home

Fear and Anxiety

While as we have discussed, fear and trauma fit into the broader picture of psychological responses to loss and grief, anxiety remains a state of unease, a feeling of worry or disquiet. Anxiety is much more of a daily occurrence with vision loss. A vast majority of clients joining discussion groups identify frustration, Anxiety and fear, as typical responses to vision loss. How to manage these responses remains a key to success.

Fear as defined by the Oxford English Dictionary is 'an unpleasant emotion caused by the threat of danger, pain, or harm' Anxiety, a sub-set of fear, 'is a feeling of worry, nervousness or unease of something with an uncertain outcome.' When it is not a direct fear for our life, the tiger about to pounce or the plane to crash, fear is actually the foundation of most of our human responses of worry and anxiety. It is therefore worth examining fear before proceeding further.

Understanding Fear

Fear stems from our survival instincts, our essential DNA. The concept of flight or fight is quite well known and understood. However, the concept of 'freeze', the third component of our primary response, the need to stay still to survive, to be camouflaged for safety, is not so frequently mentioned, but forms a large part of our response to vision loss. We will all have heard of becoming paralysed with fear and many report this occurs with sight loss. It was quite surprising to find, that when I mentioned 'freeze' as a natural response to losing sight, that most clients said, 'Ah, so that's what is happening, now I understand why I feel I can't move!'

These primary responses have been identified as coming from our 'Reptilian Brain'. And while this terminology is no longer espoused by neuroscientists,[91] this part of our brain is responsible for primary regulatory functions: heart rate and breathing etc. It is supposed to be responsible for instinctive behaviours such as acts of self-preservation, aggression, nurture, dominance, territoriality, ritual and also reproductive responses. All are designed to assist us distinguishing between threatening and non-threatening behaviours.

Of great interest and even surprise is the fact that we are born with only two primary fears. They are, fear of falling and of loud noise.[92] This suggests the remainder are learnt, cultural or environmental and therefore can be un-learnt.

Some common fears include fear of spiders, social settings, public speaking, loneliness, blindness, poverty, sickness and animals.

When these fears become irrational or an aversion to something, they are called phobias. Example include aerophobia (flying), agoraphobia (open spaces), mysophobia (germs), claustrophobia (small spaces), astraphobia (thunder), arachnophobia (spiders).

Fears concerning non-life threatening situations aren't real, they are regarded as illusions and don't exist except in our minds. They are responses to ideas that we've created from things we thought were true but actually were not, for example fears of the dark.[93]

Fear is of course, not necessarily bad. Fear, worry and anxiety can make you do things and find solutions, they can make you prepare for the worst and prevent things happening.

Understanding Anxiety

Anxieties stemming from our fears of sight loss can become deep-seated and habitual, often leading to further incapacity and illness. Everyone experiences anxiety in some form and at some time. At least one in 20 people experience general anxiety.[94]

Anxiety can be good, but becomes a concern when it feels uncontrollable, is excessive, persistent — always there, intrusive and seemingly impairing your ability to get on with your daily life. (See the section called Identifying Early Signs Of Depression, below.)

To find out if you might have an anxiety problem, ask yourself these questions:

- Are these anxieties and worries constantly in your head, repeating themselves?
- Have anxiety and worry taken over your emotions and you feel out of control?
- Are you hating uncertainty and wanting to know of solutions and cures and of what is going to happen in the future?
- Are you feeling so restless, keyed-up and on edge that you can't settle quietly and relax?
- Are you physically tense, irritated and nervy, uptight with tight muscles, stiffness and headaches?
- Are you experiencing sleeplessness, fatigue and difficulty focusing on tasks?
- Are you procrastinating and putting off decisions that seem too difficult and overwhelming?
- Are you avoiding situations where you feel apprehensive or nervous?

You don't have to experience all of the above, but one or several may be indicators of anxiety, which you can control.

Many people coming into my support groups with vision loss

tell me they make themselves busy to give themselves 'no time to think about it!' It's a method of taking their mind off unpleasant realities. This is a classic denial and avoidance response. As noted, psychologist Hugh Mackay says, 'We make ourselves busy as a hiding place.'[95]

Making ourselves busy is not necessarily bad, but you need to be aware of the impact of such responses in terms of avoiding issues that need to be faced. Adopting a mindfulness and problem-solving approach will be more helpful.

Mindfulness

The concept of mindfulness is now widely used as an approach to understanding yourself and dealing with stress, anger and anxiety — issues common to sight loss. The Mayo Clinic defines mindfulness as a type of meditation in which you focus on being intensely aware of what you're sensing and feeling in the moment, without interpretation or judgment.[96] The Headspace organisation's definition is similar: 'the quality of being present and fully engaged with whatever we're doing at the moment, free from distraction or judgment, and aware of our thoughts and feelings without getting caught up in them. We train in this moment-to-moment awareness through meditation, allowing us to build the skill of mindfulness so that we can then apply it to everyday life. In teaching the mind to be present, we are teaching ourselves to live in the present, taking a breath, not beholden to reactive thoughts and feelings, wishing for change, or the past.' (Headspace recommends using their app.)[97]

Proponents of mindfulness say that it is not a temporary state of mind found with meditation, but a way of living that permits us to live in the present moment, not the past or future. By becoming aware of unpleasant thoughts and emotions associated with challenges, stress, anger and anxiety, we become more thoughtful and rational in our response.

The concepts of neuro-plasticity and our brain's capacity to change, as earlier referred to, once again resurface as relevant in understanding mindfulness. Proponents say mindfulness meditation does not only change our mind set and perspective; it actually can change the shape of our brain's neuro pathways. Generalised neuroimaging meditation studies found that eight weeks of mindfulness meditation also changes our brains, rewiring them towards more positive thoughts and emotions.[98]

People who incorporate mindfulness into their lives often report heightened levels of happiness, patience, acceptance and compassion, as well as lower levels of stress, frustration and sadness. Studies conducted by US North-eastern University found that three weeks of Headspace mindfulness meditation increased compassion by 23 per cent and reduced aggression by 57 per cent. What's more, another study found that eight weeks of mindfulness increased positivity and wellbeing.[99]

So in practical terms, rather than dismissing your feelings by making yourself busy, or remaining stoic, learn how to observe your physical, mental and psychological state. Consider every small detail around you and expand your thoughts to write or describe the detail. You can transpose everyday actions into some sensual appreciation such as, what are your feelings about daily occurrences, warm sun, scent of flowers, wind in the trees, tastes of food drinks and so on, then celebrate these sensations.

By doing this you are heightening your sensory capabilities, just as I have discussed with responses to vision loss, smell, taste and hearing can be heightened by increased use, (neuro-plasticity).

Enhancing everyday experiences allows you to not focus on matters out of reach, for example, not being able to see things, driving, reading etc. and that our other sensory capacities can compensate for this loss. Also, in moments of panic, return to the present moment and things you can manage, for example, your own breathing and slow it down with deep breaths. Meditation can be based upon mantras, prayer, or your breathing and a central point of your body, such as your navel. To learn meditation, find a teacher, or use an app (such as the Headspace one) or a recorded exercise on a CD, or app.

Adopting a Problem-solving Approach: Don't Eat the Whole Elephant

If we look at anxiety practically, as an everyday event, our feelings of anxiety and frustration cause our minds to race, like a highly revving engine where problems we face, like losing vision, overwhelm us. Not only does this scramble our decision-making process, but it takes up much of our energy. There may appear to be too many issues, too much to handle and when you can't see clearly, all seem overwhelming. While mindfulness discussed above is highly relevant, in facing daily issues we tend to lump every issue into a feeling of helplessness, of becoming out of control, of frustration, saying: I can't! I can't handle this! I can't cope! This merging of issues into one feeling is the elephant!

If you were asked to eat an elephant, of course, you might say,

'I can't!' It's too large. However, if you were to try, you might start with the tail, part of an ear or part of a leg, or something little, of course. This is exactly what problem solving is about, dividing things into small parts.

As I discuss later in this chapter, we must, yes, it is emphatic, 'MUST!' break down our anxieties into parts. To start with, place our worries and apprehensions into a list, preferably written, then order these into what is most or less important to you. On their own, each problem or issue has an answer. The question then becomes: Is this something I have control over? You can only solve problems that you, yes, little old you, can take action on, but this in turn raises another question: Is the problem one where I can ask someone else to assist?

With techniques of problem solving you can move to a state of relaxation, where you can identify if worry and anxiety are controlling you. For instance, do you feel that worry is controlling you, always, mostly, sometimes, hardly ever? At this point you might then identify whether this is a belief or a fact, then proceed to rate it from one to ten in order of importance, or identify what is the cause. For example, if you have just been diagnosed as having vision loss where the doctor cannot offer a cure, the question, 'Will I go blind and is there a cure?' are mostly ones of fact. But things tend to blur into one overall problem when you attempt to deal with a daily life where you can no longer drive, read clearly, watch TV or identify faces of friends, or you worry about what others think or say. Each item has its own solutions. To deal with these issues requires change and this will raise a series of ongoing frustrations because you don't know what to do. Apart from breaking down each issue into small parts, re-skilling to do things differently will also enable you to keep on coping. Naturally enough, this takes knowledge and time. Re-skilling and the patience to find answers are also a necessary part of problem solving.

Creating a List

When vision loss is recent, a whole range of thoughts and worries may be swirling around in your head. There may be so many issues arising that we feel we cannot manage them all, or find solutions so that a sense of falling out of control arises: 'Stop the world, I want to get off.'

With all problem solving, the key is to also break down and identify each worry into where and when it is happening and how does it affect you. For example, are they happening at work or at home? Do they concern your health, family, relationships, finances? What will happen in the future?

Make a list and then rate these worries in order of importance from 10 to 1 — 10 being most important — and ask yourself how often they occur. If after watching these issues for a week, ask yourself, did it occur? If it didn't, what was the impact? In this way, you might identify that some of your worries are not real or urgent. They may be issues you cannot control anyway. This will allow you to remove them from your list and therefore your thinking.

If the first problem is, well, I can't make a list, I can't see and I can't write, then use adaptive technology, a dictation machine, a family member, or a volunteer. See, already there's a solution. In creating this list, you may also feel awkward or embarrassed, hold a fear about what others might say, be afraid to be seen as weak or as a failure, and feel shy about listing them down. These reactions are quite normal. Studies confirm some people have inherited vulnerability, which includes mood disorders. You may be naturally nervous, intense and sensitive. This can be affected by environmental factors and a learned capacity to respond in a negative way. So, don't feel that this is just you being fearful. Remember, most fears are learnt.

In the above process you will be required to challenge your beliefs. You will be also asking is this a belief and is it controllable? What is the evidence supporting my belief? If your belief can be distracted by, say the phone ringing, or a friend calling over, what does this tell you? Can you distract yourself from dwelling on problems by, for example, acknowledging the little things in your life and asking what you have done successfully? Or through things such as reading, walking, music, coffee with friends? If your worrying can be distracted, then it is not uncontrollable. Write down what you think might happen if the worry is put off.

Dealing with Frustrations

Frustration is the feeling of being upset or annoyed if you can't change things, or if progress or fulfilment of a task is prevented, and it is inextricably linked to vision loss. All people I met with vision loss reported frustration becoming a major part of their lives. From every task, no matter how small or infrequent, the barrier thrown up by blurred, foggy or no sight, interferes with everything.

Here is a helpful check list for dealing with frustrations:

1. Identify what is making you anxious, then take steps learning to relax in these situations. Is there another way of doing it? Is there someone you can ask to help? Do you have the contact telephone number to ring for assistance?

2. When feeling stressed by your frustrations, try to relax by slowing down the thoughts, for example, breathe in peace, breathe out stress. Yoga is good for this.

3. Diet: Eat healthily, and limit your intake of meat products and refined foods such as refined sugar and white bread. Try to eat lots of fruits and vegetables.

4. Talk politely and be open and honest. Respect other viewpoints. Do not gossip or criticise others.

5. Be around cheerful and optimistic friends who think positively about life. This nontoxic environment will encourage you to see life in a positive manner and make it easier to cope with stress. It is best to avoid being around people who are always angry, who tend to always have a negative outlook on life and who often criticise others.

6. Remember, you can do whatever you wish if you have a problem-solving attitude.

7. Treat yourself regularly: have a massage, try yoga, meditation, aromatherapy or any alternative therapy.

8. Remove obstacles by seeing the problems as an opportunity of improving your skills or sense of self.

Identifying Early Signs of Depression

Many of us worry that we may be depressed, believing this to be an admission of weakness. In Australia, it's estimated that

45 per cent of people will experience a mental health condition in their lifetime. In any one year, around a million Australian adults have depression, and over three million have anxiety.[100] Based upon the diverse client responses in my groups and my own experience over 50 years, sadness may be experienced sometimes, but depression brings about a much stronger sense of hopelessness. When you are depressed, the world can become just a monotone grey, or black. It is hard to motivate yourself, or even get out of bed in the morning. However, my main message here is that everyone is different, there are numerous causes of vision loss and care must be taken to understand the individual's circumstances

Here are some of the early warning signs of depression:

- Sleep patterns: trouble falling asleep, waking frequently during the night and not feeling rested, or waking early. Alternatively, feeling exhausted after work, skipping meals or remaining in bed all weekend.
- Lack of motivation: no longer enjoying things you once did. The thought of doing them is tiring.
- Loss of pleasure in doing things you used to enjoy, social or physical — called Anhedonia. Lack of enjoyment with others or touch, food or sex. A feeling of detachment.
- A short fuse: little things upset you, a feeling they won't get better.
- Feelings everything is difficult: with everyday tasks, feeling you are working very hard, lack of energy.
- Loss of appetite, or conversely, eating as a distraction.

- Lack of patience: snapping at others. Does this happen all the time?
- Heightened anxiety, worry or being self-critical, noting that increased anxiety might make you 'jittery'. Are you taking shallow breaths?
- Saying you 'don't care' as an attempt to avoid painful feelings. Is this happening regularly?
- Wanting to spend more time alone, lack of energy or self-esteem.
- Lack of concentration, trying to solve unanswerable questions, dwelling in the past or worrying.

If you notice these changes, or someone points them out to you, it may be a good idea to reach out for help. As referred to in my discussion of Adjustment Disorder Chapter 1, being aware of solutions and holding hope that your situation can improve will prevent you sliding into denial and avoidance, even depression. Going to a psychologist or group therapy, making some lifestyle changes, and possibly even taking medication, keeps depression from taking over.[101]

The Need to Become Assertive

As we start to move forward and begin to grapple with many of the feelings and responses to vision loss mentioned above and take up services to begin re-skilling ourselves, we will have to start asking for help, services and answers. In other words, we have to be assertive. This is where we become confident and forceful, no longer passively accepting our fate and asking what can I do now to improve my situation? Some steps include:

- With advice, prepare and plan what you want to do, being aware this might take longer than before your vision was impaired, and bearing in mind what is possible when it comes to asking others for help.
- Think through the rights and responsibilities of each person in the situation. Not doing this and making yourself the focus of attention becomes the basis for aggression.
- Be clear about what you are asking for and its implications.
- Gather information and know your options and rights. Talking to others, or joining a peer social or discussion group, is very helpful here.
- Identify the skills you bring and the contribution you can make.

Improving Self-esteem

As we recover from the shock of facing vision loss and begin to move forward, we need to think about who we were before vision loss. What were the qualities and values you held which made you who you are? Perhaps you were at the top of your work, saw yourself as capable and now vision loss has knocked the 'stuffing' out of you? Well, it time to start to rebuild your skills. All the people I have spoken with and read about who rebuild their lives say, 'persistence' becomes a key word.

However, if in the course of undertaking this reflection, you believe you have no skills or capabilities, nothing to offer, it will perhaps suggest a depressive state where you need to seek further professional support. But remember, everyone has good qualities and climbing a mountain always starts at the bottom.

Self-esteem means, confidence in one's own worth and abilities, self-respect. Ask yourself the following questions and write down the answers. This is not about achieving a top score; it's about identifying things you do or say. If you feel you can't answer one, you are not a failure. The list is to let you evaluate how you think about yourself. Remember, everyone is different.

- What are the things you value about yourself?
- What are the things that happen to you and make you feel good?
- What do you think are your skills and talents?
- Do you help others? In what way?
- What are the attitudes you see in others that help you feel good?

As mentioned, the above questions are not a rating system. You will be able to think of an answer and feel positive about this. Consider whether you might need to change things. The answers will also tell you if there are areas in which you might want to change.

Now, ask yourself some more questions, to help identify how you feel about yourself, whether you are allowing your needs to be overridden and whether you might need to become more assertive:

Can you think of a time when it was difficult to express your needs? For example:

- In refusing an invitation,
- Stopping someone from being rude,

- Saying 'no' to unreasonable demands,
- In asking for assistance/help,
- Not wanting to hurt someone's feelings,
- Feeling the need to avoid conflict.

If you find that you are giving in to one or all of the above requests or feelings, you are not expressing your needs and perhaps you need to become more assertive. It is important to remember that being assertive is balancing your rights and needs with those of others. Overriding others' needs is viewed as aggression. Allowing your needs to be overridden is being passive.

If you feel you have to support everyone, be kind, or go along because you don't want to make a fuss, be a nuisance etc., you are part of the passive/stoic personality I referred to earlier. When you can't say 'no' yet you still feel you have more important issues to deal with, then this will indicate you are allowing your needs to be overridden. Perhaps you need to work on becoming more assertive. In other chapters in this book I discuss why vision loss makes us withdraw and some of the many skills we can acquire which enable us to remain independent, assertive and confident.

Now, after all this, even for having read and thought about this chapter, it's time to praise yourself. You actually can do things differently to the way you did them before. As T. S. Eliot wrote: 'Praise is the enemy of cynicism and depression. It is the Engine of self-esteem. It has the Power to change a life, change a culture, and therefore a country.'

9

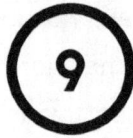

Attitudes with Partial Sight

'The method for finding your way is much alike both for the blind and the sighted. In an unfamiliar place, it may be necessary to ask for directions. If the directions are correct and complete, this solves the problem. If not, a request for more information may be made. This is how all of us learn how to get where we want to go.'

Dr Kenneth Jernigan, US NFB former President.

'Although we love the idea of choice, our culture almost worships it. We seek refuge in the familiar and the comfortable.'

Hugh Mackay, psychologist

Feeling a Fake or a Fraud

Time and time again in facilitating discussion groups with partially sighted people, I've heard comments like this: 'I feel a fake coming here!' Or 'I feel a fraud, my eyesight is not that bad!' Those people felt as I once did, that because you still have some residual sight, you are not entitled to, or should not 'take up', vision loss services, government support, or use white canes or other aids. Often when struggling on in denial of their low vision handicap they still said, 'I'm not ready yet!' Perhaps that last comment explains why. People have to be ready to take up change and accept that such changes are necessary. Once their experiences are 'normalised' all will be okay.

There are really two reasonable responses to feeling a 'fake':

First, there is no correct time to accept services; our vision loss experiences are all different. We do not have to admit to a vision disability if we can manage successfully. (See 'Using Remaining Sight Successfully', below.)

Even people who lose one eye can experience significant trauma, fearing loss of the remaining eye. They need time to adjust to a visual field reduced from 180 degrees to 130 degrees. (As we get older we might experience difficulty with night blindness, visual acuity, the sharpness of vision, reduced peripheral vision, depth perception and colour vision.) Restrictions on driving don't apply until acuity diminishes, for example the visual acuity in the remaining eye is 6/12 or better, with or without correction and the visual field in the remaining eye has a horizontal extent of at least 110 degrees within 10 degrees above and below the horizontal mid-line.[102] There should be no reason why you cannot function normally with one eye. However, it was quite amazing the number of clients who came to discussion groups when really, their sight, at least in respect to their remaining acuity, was still excellent.

Second, where is the tipping point? That is the point where it just doesn't make sense to continue struggling with poor sight. This is the great challenge. Sight is so important to our sensory perception that we find it very hard to stop using our eyes to look at things. Even before a doctor or optometrist says you shouldn't drive or he/she can't help with new glasses, the time to change to aids such as white canes and smart audio devices can be assessed by any one of the following:

- You start making mistakes in reading and recognising objects, and start apologising for these mistakes.
- You start to trip, even fall.
- You have difficulty seeing street numbers, glass doors, lifts.
- You feel embarrassed about not seeing faces and use ruses to guess identity.
- Corrected spectacles don't help; you constantly peer at text.
- You struggle with reading and withdraw from reading books and newspapers.
- You stop going out, and have poor night vision.
- You experience degrees of fear, frustration and anger.
- You become reluctant to socialise and no longer maintain communications with friends.

Some people struggle on using magnifying glasses, or computer screen magnification reading letter by letter, slowly and painstakingly to a point where it is surely self-defeating. As sight diminishes slowly, we can become like the frog in slowly boiling water, we don't jump out until it is too late. We may not be able to compare ourselves with other people with vision impairment who are far more capable and productive. Only you, the person experiencing vision loss, can tell when you're at the tipping point, but in pulling back because 'it's too hard' we also cut ourselves off from finding more effective solutions such as asking for help. Adam from Victoria, a participant in a discussion group in 2016, told of how following a massive stroke and resulting partial vision loss, he felt he could not resume work or a normal life. He said at the conclusion of the group, 'Our discussions gave me the light bulb moment, that what was stopping me going back to work was that I didn't know how to explain my vision loss and ask for help from my work colleagues. I didn't want to appear helpless. I gained the confidence to realise how I could ask for help only when and how I needed it and avoid other workmates becoming afraid I was generally helpless!' Adam now works full time and travels around the world.

Even Successful Painters and Writers Can Be Vision Impaired

Vision impairment is no barrier to artistic endeavours. Alice, an artist from Sydney with macular degeneration, said in 2012 that in coming to terms with her grief, 'I had to de-clutter my home and also my mind. I gave away all my etchings and photos to stop thinking about what I could no longer do and reduced the number of brushes to three, then simplified all my tubes of colours, placing them into three tins with red, blue and yellow lids!' Alice still successfully paints and wins competitions, but her art is different to the way she did so before.

A blind man in Britain creates 3D tactile collage paintings from materials with different textures. Famous artists such as Claude Monet who had cataracts and Edgar Degas with retinal disease for his last fifty years, were vision impaired. Degas turned to sculpture as a more friendly tactile medium. Some more recent artists include Eşref Armağan, a Turkish artist born without eyes; Keith Salmon, a visually impaired artist working in Ayrshire, Scotland; and Michael Naranjo, a blind Native American sculptor who lost eyesight in Vietnam. Some books that discuss vision loss and techniques for painting are, Elisabeth Salzhauer Axel's Art Beyond Sight: A Resource Guide to Art, Creativity, and Visual Impairment, and John Kennedy's Drawing and the Blind: Perceptions to Touch, which focuses on the ways in which the blind, both young and old, can perceive pictures.

Some famous writers had partial sight or were blind. James Joyce, author of Ulysses, spent 17 years writing Finnegans Wake using a small sliver of sight and writing with crayons. The British author Aldous Huxley was vision impaired for his last 20 years and the Argentinian writer, Jorge Luis Borges still wrote, despite his eventual total blindness.

Partial sight does have a slower pathway to acceptance. Not only do we continue to use remaining sight, but the natural and most powerful habit of looking, is hard to break, but break it we must if we are to use our other faculties and place our trust in technology.

Using Remaining Sight Successfully

While we have discussed in this book the need to adapt to vision loss and change our way of doing things, there is also a need for those with partial sight loss to understand the extent of retained useable sight and use it, provided no eye strain or harm takes place.

As previously mentioned, the vast majority (79 per cent) of those with vision loss may retain some useable sight, and even a majority of the 18 per cent of people who are legally blind, might retain some sight helpful for orientation. For example, many of those with macular degeneration, the second largest cause of vision loss, having lost their central vision and a capacity to focus on fine work and read etc., often don't realise that they still may have significant useable areas of peripheral field vision. Those with cataracts whose sight is foggy, will need to rely upon touch. People with glaucoma, or affected by stroke, can also have patches of useable sight. Visual field training may be required for you to be effective, although you can train yourself to rotate, or move your eyes, or look to the side or upwards to see things. Such movements may make you look a little odd, but remember: what others might think of you doesn't matter, it's what you need to do for maintaining independence that is most important.

When you think of using your remaining sight, just remember people who are totally blind continue with tasks and hobbies that most believe is impossible. For example, knitting, sewing, crochet, cooking, woodwork, motor repairs (See Chapter 18), where people say they do all this from either memory and being very well organised. One of my discussion group members, who is totally blind, rebuilt a Corvette sports car, while others work on rebuilding combustion engines. A man now completely blind with retinitis pigmentosa, undertakes all mechanical work for his Torana racing cars and his son's go-karts. Many women said they could no longer crochet, but a totally blind woman cheerily told our group she continued to crochet using 'touch and muscle memory'. Yes! It's not easy, and you might have to ask for help along the way, but you can do it if you have the will.

With some diseases, such as retinitis pigmentosa, too much light is not helpful for the retina, and some research now indicates that 'blue light' is also harmful for macular degeneration as well. If you find that you are struggling to see, taking a long time to read, or in doing so you are getting headaches, it may be better to seek professional advice and move to using adaptive audio and voice recognition technology as the better option. However, by working with a person skilled in ophthalmic support, you can train yourself to use remaining areas of sight more effectively. There is also a range of equipment such as CCTV scanners, smartphone apps, monoculars or other gadgets that may assist.

The broad principles of using remaining sight include the three 'Bs' of making things 'bigger, bolder and brighter'. For example:

1. Bigger. Make letters and writing bigger or use magnifying glasses.
2. Bolder. Use contrasting stronger colours such as deep black letters, or cutting boards that provide contrast to your kitchen bench.
3. Brighter. Use better lighting, lamps, appropriate light bulbs or reduce glare. LED lighting is popular.

Using vision rehabilitation services and training usually provided by an occupational therapist, can provide you with techniques that can help you accomplish the bigger, bolder, brighter principles. For example, making print larger, using optical and electronic magnifiers, changing computer screen contrast to reduce glare, using large print or tactile aids such as puff paint or stick-on raised dots, installing better lighting, using contrasting colours and smart technology are part of these solutions. (See Chapter 16, Independence in the Home.)

Functioning with Reduced Sight

Here are some further tips to make the most of whatever sight you may have. See also Chapters 15–17 for further tips.

1. Use your remaining senses — touch, taste, smell and hearing — for better effect. For example, if identifying herbs for cooking, smell can be effective, so you don't have to read the label. You can use your feet to feel differences in surfaces, for example walking from carpeted areas to tiled areas.
2. Use tactile markers, or audio reading devices for example, in handling medicines safely and other storage equipment such as pill dispensers.
3. Improve organisation and planning. De-clutter your home and work places. For example, keep pantry, bench tops, floor areas, and backyard workshop areas clean and ordered. (See Chapter 16, Independence in the Home.)
4. De-clutter your mind, for example reduce anxiety, the grief of hanging onto sight and a former world.

5. Educate family and others that you can do things, but that you might be slower or different in the way you carry out the task than in the past.
6. Take advantage of rehabilitation support, such as orientation and mobility and occupational therapy and ophthalmic services.
7. Switch over to using smart technology and apps that read text.

So much of our capacity and daily functions depend upon our vision. Our sight feeds in information, which our brain processes in a split second. We do not even think, but are nevertheless aware of our surroundings and automatically respond. For example, in walking out the door, without hesitation, a sighted person's peripheral vision might spot the note you wrote, see your door keys, spot your jacket hung over a chair, see the switch to turn the light off and take a quick look to see the gas is turned off, and do this in their stride, in a second or two. However, for someone with vision loss, each of the above steps will now require more time and perhaps be dealt with in separate steps, need a greater concentration of thoughts to remember where things are, perhaps a number of attempts to feel for keys, jacket or light switch, and then walk to the stove to check the gas is turned off. These steps take conscious mental effort, adding to fatigue and frustration, and allowing more time to do daily tasks is essential.

Best Practice for Vision Impairment

Your inability to identify people and not see faces, or give a normal wave of recognition across a room, or street, is one of the most confronting effects of early vision loss.[103] As previously noted, feelings of frustration through social isolation can quickly lead to anxiety, resentment, anger or depression. The simple but sometimes difficult solution to apply when you can no longer identify faces is to say, 'My eyesight is not so good now, can you please give your name from now on when we meet?'

Another approach mostly resisted in the early stages of sight loss, is to wear an ID badge that states, 'I've got low vision', or 'I use the ID small white cane'. It is only when we recognise the above requirements as important, that we arrive at a point where we can say to ourselves, 'It doesn't matter what others think!' Or 'I need to do what is best for me'. At that point, we can move on to another level. We commence regaining control over feelings of helplessness, and be strong enough, for example, to ask others to give their names when speaking. This places us back on a level footing. Yes, it does work!

Best Practice for Sighted Friends

It is simple for people with sight to give their name when introducing themselves. If you want to shake hands, wait until the person with vision impairment puts their hand out where you can then grasp it.

For sighted people, if you know someone has vision impairment, ask if they might like some assistance.

Some Impacts on Health

Our struggle with the physical changes and associated emotions can have a major effect on our health and outlook.

You may have expectations that you should be better or more capable than what you feel you are, or that your personality has changed. 'I don't want to make a fool of myself!' You may feel shy, embarrassed become withdrawn or even depressed.

Many, many people with vision loss therefore report that they are 'so tired'. 'I just feel exhausted!' It's an important fact to note that our brain is only approximately 2 per cent of our body weight,[104] but it normally takes about 20 per cent of our energy.[105] So if you are using your brain and memory much more because of vision loss — as we do! — then increased tiredness/fatigue are to be expected. As a consequence, we have to take longer to do things, to plan and prepare more. Don't let yourself get caught in unplanned and perhaps stressful situations.

But on a day-to-day basis, having to think where everything is, or wonder 'How am I going to get down the street?' can be all-consuming, creating anxiety or feelings of stress that affect our ability to think clearly. Even panic attacks and hyper-ventilation can occur. Effective problem-solving techniques are essential. (See Chapter 8, Dealing with Worry, Anxiety and Stress.)

With all the thinking now required, we may even feel loss of memory as our thoughts become overloaded. We may experience headaches, stiff necks, back aches because of our changed posture as we now stoop to see things clearly, loss of appetite, or sleeplessness. It is a fact that with loss of vision, our body clock can be also affected, a condition called Non-24-Hour Sleep-Wake Disorder, which may require medication, but consult your medical professional.

In attempting not to give in to the above feelings and in our desire to succeed, to 'fight' it and not give up, there is a tendency to push ourselves to extremes at work, school or home. Sometimes we may start a demanding exercise regime, look for cures and take food or vitamin supplements.

The above reactions, if not understood and recognised as our natural response not to fail, can hold us back from coming to terms with our disability and block us from taking up solutions.

Government Supports

I can't tell you how often clients coming into my discussion groups after visiting their medical professional or service provider, said, 'I don't know what supports there are, no one tells you!' This view is supported by Blind Citizens Australia (BCA), which states that 'it has become clear that service providers and professionals who diagnose vision loss do not always provide their clients with appropriate information and referrals'. In response, BCA has created state-by-state 'Toolkits'. I've provided a summary below.[106]

The best advice for International readers is to contact their blind and vision impaired support organisations to ascertain what Governmental, financial and rehabilitative supports exist.

Summary of Key Supports in Australia

- Disability Support Pension — Blind (age 65 or less) — is not means tested unlike the ordinary DSP
- Aged Pension — Blind (over 65years) — is not means tested, unlike the ordinary Aged Pension
- Vision Impaired Travel Pass — for Public Transport in all states

- Taxi Subsidy Schemes (half price with a cap, varying between states and obtain Interstate vouchers) — now under review in some states because of the National Disability Insurance Scheme (NDIS); in Victoria it is means tested
- Energy, water and phone supplements
- Concessions on local government house rates
- Reduced car registrations and parking concessions
- The National Disability Insurance Scheme (NDIS) under 65 years
- My Aged Care (MAC) — over 65 years

There are many more benefits, including travel assistance, education and training, too numerous to list here.

One major benefit in Australia is the Companion Card (www. companioncard.org.au, Tel: 1800 650 611, National Relay Service: 13 36 77). It is issued by state governments, and is now nationwide. This entitles you to take a companion (who doesn't have to be a relative) free of charge to most events, including the theatre, movies, sport events, galleries and on public transport. While it is easier to obtain this if you are legally blind, this status is not essential. The primary test is, can you safely attend a venue on your own, taking into account evacuation safety procedures required in the event of fire? If your answer is no, then you may be eligible. This card contributes significantly to improved social and community participation. If you are legally blind, a doctor, authorised social worker or occupational therapist is able to assist you to fill in the form and sign it.

First Steps

The message of Orientation and Mobility specialists and of most Peers who succeed with re-skilling themselves, is to take small steps. Consider the following:

Use the supports offered by service organisations that specialise in understanding the needs of vision impairment.

Don't be passive just making one call and then sitting back to wait. Service contact is meant to be within three days. If you don't get a response, be ASSERTIVE! After a reasonable time, ring back or send an email, that is assuming you can use your email system, or get someone to send this for you. After two attempts and you get no response,, escalate your call to the supervisor or team manager. there are also established complaints systems. Use this if you feel you need to.

You only need one good friend. Many people worry about losing friends, but if friends don't want to be with you, see this as their problem not yours. As a client said, 'I got rid of my toxic friends!'

- Actively gain knowledge and information on what is possible, what directions you should take and what technology helps.
- Join a discussion group, or client support group. A peer support program in Australia called the Quality Living Program conducted by Vision Australia, can provide you with an overview of what is out there and allow you to discuss emotional responses with others in similar situations.
- Get professionals such as Orientation and Mobility (O&M) specialists to talk to your family and allow them to understand what low vision means, why a white cane might be necessary and how to be a 'sighted guide' and other techniques.

- Get adaptive technology specialists (ATS) to assist and train you to use technology.
- Get an occupational therapist (OT) to come to your home and identify tasks you struggle with, likely dangers and identify solutions.
- Have simulation glasses, which mimic what eye diseases look like so that others around you can understand what you can and can't see.
- Develop assertiveness skills and sighted guide techniques. Use words that gain best effect. For example, if someone tries to take over by doing the cooking or washing, or grabs your arm to push you around, say, 'Thank you for asking, but I'm OK!' or 'Stop! I'd like you to assist this way!' or 'Thanks, if I need some help I'll ask for it!'
- Be assertive in setting up systems in your home which suit you, like organising the fridge, pantry, computer, etc., and ask for others to respect and support your system.
- Don't be bullied into moving to a care home. It is important to understand that vision loss itself should not be the reason to go into aged or supportive care unless you really want to. People with vision loss can retain independence by doing things differently.
- Put your needs first. If you need to use a cane for safety when you go out — use it! Or if you feel too embarrassed, keep it folded up in your bag. However, realise that the white cane has a stigma of blindness which other family members may feel embarrassed about. They need to understand and be educated on how a cane helps you as a navigational tool. In

some families, ethnic or cultural values may create resistance, or children may not like their mum or dad to have a cane.

- You will have to become an 'educator' of others so they understand your needs.

As hard as it is to believe, you don't have to have sight to do most things. For example, touch can replace sight, using smartphones — they talk to us and we can use voice recognition to activate apps on the phone, or to ring someone on your contact list.

Understand that by using touch, you can do almost anything, using tactile markers, accessible equipment and aids.

Realise that technology with audio now offers many solutions. In particular, voice recognition apps or devices such as Google Home, Alexa and Apple products are life-changing. Accessible software for computers such as JAWS and NVDA enable text recognition and speech.

Now, believe it, there is another life after vision loss and you can find it!

(10)

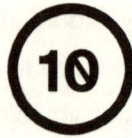

Accepting You Will Be Different

'I wasted a lot of emotional energy thinking of what I could not do rather than the extraordinary amount I was doing.'

Jane Poulsen, MD, blind physician

'When I discover who I am, I'll be free.'

Ralph Ellison, The Invisible Man

'Normal is not something to aspire to, it's something to get away from.'

Jodie Foster, actress and director

The Reality Check: It's All about Attitude

Years ago, while still farming and hardened by a series of drawn-out struggles which included finding out I had incurable eye disease, I came to regard myself like the tormented figure in Norwegian Edvard Munch's The Scream. The painting depicts a haunted face, denuded of all qualities and surrounded by a bleak and desolate landscape — desperate, frantic, crying out, muffled by impervious bubbles of the psyche. I was repulsed when I first saw this dramatic painting, but later with my increasing frustrations I related to its expressions of tormented emotion and began to feel great affinity with its mood and meaning. Like the subject, I felt trapped in a bubble where my screams of emotional desperation could not be heard. Even the place for my last act was identified. A spot facing my favourite view, northwards over beautiful blue Mount Tarongo where in summer I had marvelled over towering Wagnerian thunderheads whose turbulent plumes reached the jet stream some 10,000 metres high to form supernatural anvils. Walhalla, I thought, would be a blessed relief, a place for peaceful release from all my struggles. When I found out another life was possible, that I could retrain myself and that I could move away from my sorrow, I realised vision loss was not the end of the world, just another one of life's hurdles. So by way of this reality check, I gained hope sufficient to quell my turbulent depressive emotions and move on.

If people who are totally blind can reach the top of their profession, or even just manage their lives successfully, then so can you. It's a message very hard to convey to those who, just beginning their vision loss journey, remain in a low state. However, life does, it can and it will, actually get better through self-belief, a confidence coming from re-skilling, knowing life can be different and that difference is something to be proud of.

As Jane Fonda says, 'The most incredible beauty and the most satisfying way of life come from affirming your own uniqueness.'

Accepting Responsibility

I found that a very large part of coming to terms with vision loss, its accompanying frustration and stress, involves acknowledging our emotions. We may wish that things could be better, or that someone, not me, should do something. However, we must take responsibility for ourselves! We might feel that because our assumed capacities have been so denied by sight loss, someone else 'should do something about it because we can't!' Why don't 'politicians do something?' Or 'Why don't doctors find a cure?' Or 'why don't blind agencies do something?' Or 'Why doesn't my family understand what I'm going through?'

Well, maybe there is a fundamental truth which is hard to come to terms with in our early grief. Isn't it our responsibility to assert our own cause? Then, why don't we, not others, do something about it? For example, talk to others, write a diary or your memoirs, join support groups or community organisation like Probus, or, most importantly, learn new skills with technology and give ourselves the capacity to move forward. In doing so, cast our old self aside and say 'to Hell with what others might say or think!' Erik Weihenmayer, says, the aim so to 'make blindness part of you, like having brown hair or green eyes, or being tall or short, to give it a place and make it part of you'.[107]

Heidi from Victoria, blind mother of four, said, 'I found it essential to understand that the world doesn't spin around me! It is our responsibility to take the steps to re-skill and re-train ourselves to become capable, independent and confident again. You struggle everyday — missing out, yet understanding that this is actually part of acceptance.'[108]

Accepting our disability means that we take for granted vision loss as just another part of our complex humanity.

It stands to reason then that we should not gild the lily. If you have recently been diagnosed with any of the myriad diseases that result in progressive or sudden sight loss, you may naturally be anxious or fearful of blindness and what it will mean for you! Steve Kelley writes, 'Instead of motivating you to seek guidance or resources, the fear of losing your sight may prove debilitating.'[109] As noted in Chapter 8, it can make you freeze with fear, or anxiety, not knowing where to go for guidance. However, we cannot change a fundamental truth. Transition and rehabilitation with vision loss are not easy; change may take a long time, perhaps years, but in the end, responsibility does rest with us.

How Long Does it Take?

The answer to this frequently asked question is 'It all depends on you!' Some people have a natural resilience, a positive personality, which enables them to not worry too much. Others, being introverted and sensitive, are held back by sadness and spend years grieving. I found that when people were told that solutions were possible, they quickly changed and moved on to a new way of doing things. In all honesty, if we think about it, we may never 'get over it', it's all about displacing it. Research by the American Foundation for the Blind (AFB) in the USA confirms the average time to adjust to sight loss is seven years. But it need not take so long. When revealing this fact to my discussion groups, there was often an audible exclamation, 'Ah, now I'm not being slow, or dumb'. As noted, the earlier we accept change and re-skill ourselves, the sooner we regain our life and cast the shadow of grief aside. We can draw upon our own life's experience to do this. In the end, to accept who we are, disabilities and all, means we are comfortable in our own skin and confident.

Ask yourself, What steps can I take to improve my situation? Often the answer is as simple as picking up the phone.

In the greater disability diaspora, our capacity to accept and adjust is part of our amazing human spirit. To go on when we are as scared as hell, like Jacob Bronowski's pilot in The Ascent of Man. It is, according to Bronowski, part of man's essential and unique psyche and we can accept this. As Erik Weihenmayer says, 'If you can learn to push your body, your brain isn't far behind.'[110]

Peer Support Networks

According to psychiatrists, 'social support is essential for maintaining physical and psychological health. The harmful consequences of poor social support and the protective effects of good social support in mental illness have been well documented ... Social support may moderate genetic and environmental vulnerabilities and confer resilience to stress.' [111]

For over 30 years, Australian blind agencies have conducted peer support groups providing emotional support for those experiencing vision loss. Described by participants as 'life changing', these discussion groups remain instrumental in skill development, self-empowerment and confidence building. By this process these groups 'normalise' vision disability and overcome natural tendencies for withdrawal and isolation.

After initially resisting joining a group discussion, following the eight-week program, clients have said:

Lynette, 'I'm inspired by everybody. I found it all so special in our own certain way. I feel more confident, more vocal!'

Chris, 'I feel very privileged. I feel a different person, more confident, more independent. We spoke of assertiveness and this helped me in that area!'

Kerry, 'I'm more independent, feel like I'm starting a new life. Gaining confidence and finding that I can do things again!'

Jim, 'Everybody has admitted they feel frustrated and at times angry. The whole session has been an enormous enlightenment to me!'

Helen, 'When we get the opportunity like this just to see how others are coping with it, it's just really great!'

Peter, 'I've realised that it doesn't matter how long you're blind for, you will always have the same problem. It doesn't change if it's been a month or a year. I also noticed that from the first day, everyone seems happier. When I first started there was a lot of sadness still. That's changed. It's sad that it's ending!'[112]

Mostly, in our defeated state when first confronted with vision loss, we feel we can no longer cope, let alone have the required assertiveness skills to do this. We may not want to even talk about this. We may not believe, or have the knowledge that we can find practical solutions to our everyday problems. As a discussion group client said, 'I was a little depressed when I attended my first session but on meeting others, I felt better and it's nice to make contact with others with vision loss. I've been uplifted!' In another group, Paul said, 'When I began to lose my sight, I found the whole world the same but darker, I challenged friends to play golf at midnight. I didn't think I needed to use a cane and three times I nearly ended up on someone's car bonnet before I realised something had to change!'

Broadly speaking, peer support occurs when people provide knowledge, experience, emotional, social or practical help to each other. People with a similar disability come together as a group, which may take a number of forms, such as peer mentoring, reflective listening, sharing experience and skills. The facilitator to preferably have lived, family, or relevant professional experience. Groups can meet in person, by phone or online with the essential principle that they are all equal.[113]

I make sure to encourage participants to identify with and accept the topics they wish to talk about, thus gaining ownership of their program.

To generate discussion, I often ask, 'Tell me, how has your life changed since vision loss?' Or 'Since your vision loss started, what are you finding difficult?' If a participant doesn't want to talk, is upset or crying, I don't press them to answer. Participants are not under pressure. Often many are so pleased to talk about what they are feeling that it is if a dam has burst as they tell of their pent up emotions. For many it is the first time they will have talked about how they feel. This atmosphere of openness encourages those who are too shy or upset to start speaking and, in its simplest terms, there lies the key which permits us to move forward.

Getting Started

Many Orientation and Mobility Specialists advise, 'Go slowly, take small steps!' For example, just learning how to get around your home and to the front gate, or letter box, is enough for first steps. Later, to a nearby shop or bus stop, then down town, and so on. Remember, be kind to yourself.

Naturally, no one wants to be labelled as disabled, but disability is part of our humanity. However, like most really tough decisions, once you make them and push through, we wonder why it was so hard to start. As Dr Hugh Mackay says, 'But the rule seems to be that the bigger and more life-changing the decision, the less it will seem like a decision at all.'[114]

It is natural that as we carry on, our minds may be racing, feelings of panic or anxiety may unsettle us. (See Chapter 8, Dealing with Worry, Anxiety and Stress.) We are like a duck, which above water appears all calm and peaceful, but underneath, its legs, like our emotions, are thrashing furiously! You are not alone if you feel like this. Canadian doctor Jane Poulson describes these feelings well in The Doctor Will Not See You Now, 'Despite the crippling rage within me, I looked calm, cool and collected to the curious onlooker who would stop to watch my [mobility] lessons.'[115]

Once we begin to take small steps, acceptance comes when we no longer resist, fight or dwell in self-pity and regrets. It is the reality check, I am now who I am, I can't immediately change this, now let's get moving.

Steps to take include:

- The sooner we can talk about our loss, fears and grief, the sooner we can reach emotional equilibrium again.
- The sooner we learn to ask for help, the sooner we can move forward accepting that we are now different to who and what we were before.
- The sooner we go back to Grade One and commence re-skilling ourselves, the sooner we attain the capacity to move forward again.
- Accepting vision loss also means we will be doing things differently to the way we may have done so before. This should be seen as a form of enlightenment, a strength to be proud of.

What others with vision loss who have attained acceptance say is worth considering:

'I see with my mind clearly now and the darkness has disappeared! (Cheryl, Queensland — near total vision loss.)

'I realise that I've still got a brain which works and I can do things!' (Verna, Queensland — Macular Degeneration.)

'We are only as disabled as we think we are!' (Olivia, NSW — dystrophy, light perception.)

The above quotes come from those who have realised that

they can remain fully functional, use technology to maintain independence and have lost their initial shyness or reserve about saying, 'I've got bad eyesight, can you help?'

In The End, it's All about Attitude

The businessman Fletcher Jones once said, 'Don't give me first class brains, give me first class attitudes.'[116]

So as hard as it might appear, there is definitely a life after vision loss which need not be dystopian. It comes with a realisation that we can do things, but differently to the way we did them before. Like the example I referred to previously, of Barry from Queensland, who, totally blind, jumps independently as a parachutist. How does he do it? Well, not like the silly joke, 'When you feel your dog guide's lead go slack, you know he's touched the ground before you!' But as earlier reported, he uses a friend with a radio to follow him down and provide directions, and his is the story of so many others. There is no magic here, just practical common sense and by relying upon a friend, Barry happily maintains his hobby.

Similarly, marathon runners use a short strap or piece of string joined to a companion's arm to gain guidance. Blind golfers use a sighted caddy and tandem cyclists a companion called 'captain' in the front seat. Usually, high achievers rely upon a partner, companion or team to act as their guide. The blind horserider Sue Lovett said, 'My parents encouraged me to do anything!' Many other totally blind people refer to their parents' attitudes as the reason for their success. Maurice and Nick Gleeson and the Jolley family in Victoria report that, 'Their parents never said they couldn't do something just because of their lack of sight. They always encouraged them to have a go and not be limited by what they think they can't do!' Proving that blindness does not mean that you are intellectually disabled, or no longer capable.

Bernadette Jolley from Victoria was part of a family of seven children of whom four had the genetic degenerative disease of Retinitis Pigmentosa. Bernadette, whose vision at an early age was restricted to only light/dark perception said, 'Our parents allowed us to ride tricycles around the backyard. We had great fun and we were never told not to do it. How we didn't crash I don't know, but we all felt this was normal. We didn't see ourselves as any different to others and we had a lot of fun!'

Michael Hingson, from USA, also reported in his book Thunder Dog, that he, too, was not restricted by his parents, who allowed him to ride bikes, first within his home and later down the street. Michael claims this allowed him to develop his sixth sense of sound/echo-location.[117]

If change makes you different, this is not something to be afraid of either. According to ultra-marathon runner Samantha Gash, Embracing difference is also a strength and 'unless you try, you will not find this strength within you. But it is still a choice you hold. Exercising it is empowerment. In tackling so many changes, you require 'essential resilience'[118], but this comes from also knowing that you are not alone and others have succeeded before you. In facing challenges, as Melbourne man Rohit Roy, says, 'You find out you hold more strengths than you know you've got.'[119]

The essential difference is knowing you can change. Vision loss is not death, so get on with your new life; there really is one after vision loss and a very rich and full one if you want it!

PART TWO

Some Big Picture Issues

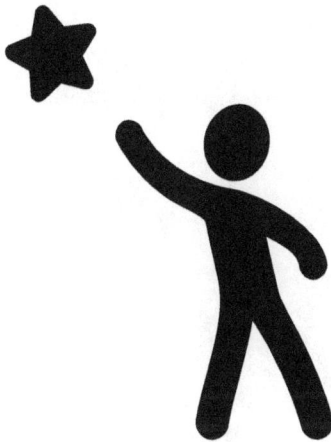

(11)

Schooling, Study and Communications

'Educating the mind without educating the heart is no education at all.'

Aristotle

'The mind is not a vessel to be filled, but a fire to be kindled.'

Plutarch

The Troubled Road Of Education

For over 14 years I conducted discussion groups for parents of children with vision loss, just parents, or for parents with vision loss who had children with or without sight loss. All these groups raised unending and complex issues about parenting, schooling, attitudes of teachers and community, of other parents, friendships, teenagers, coping and learning survival techniques. The following five Chapters summarise key issues and responses identified as a result of these discussions. I have supported many parents in tears, children in rebellion, heard heart-breaking stories of victimization and prejudice. Hopefully, at the very least, the following Chapters offer some insight and guidelines.

Beginnings With Education

When my eyesight began to fail in 1969, I regarded my future as hopeless. But then I found the Student Training and Tape Reading Section of the Royal Victorian Institute for the Blind (RVIB). Suddenly, I had hope. Here was a world of light, tolerance and radiance, where individuality was welcomed and dreams supported. The Sections leader, the redoubtable, perceptive, inspiring and compassionate Margaret Fialides, informed me I was eligible for a program called 'The Early Leaver Scheme', which provided access to University. Suddenly, I was overcome with feelings of disbelief and amazement, that a world I had thought denied was now revealed as possible.

Margaret's mantra, not too dissimilar to the Frenchman Diderot's (1749) belief of teaching directed to 'skills of the individual' was, 'Just because you are blind or vision impaired doesn't mean you don't have intelligence or intellectual capacity!' Her mantra underpinned this creative approach to learning. Does it really take nearly 200 years to effect change? Sadly, it seems yes!

In the past, along with other state and international supports, the Institute's main focus was to patronisingly typecast and shunt people with vision impairment into working in assisted workshops, woodwork factories and packaging systems, and operating telephone switchboards. To be fair, at least these were opportunities where little existed before. Behind this however, lay a belief by sighted providers that they knew what was best for the blind. In the 1940s this was the great battle of the US National Federation of the Blind (NFB), under its leader, Dr Kenneth Jernigan, to make sighted service providers listen to what the blind wanted and not presume they, the fully sighted, knew better.

By the 1970s, some rare individuals had independently established themselves in professions or in business by dint of their raw courage and perseverance, but for the most part, without higher education, such success was exceptional. There were blind social workers, barristers and academics, while a totally blind man with the support of his wife, had established a printing business. Another, the totally blind David Hume, successfully conducted his HR recruitment business. Otherwise at that time, employment outside protected workshops was a barren landscape for people with total blindness.

Margaret's revolutionary concept was based upon a simple system where volunteers were organised to read onto tape the books and other course materials required for tertiary studies, including law textbooks of 200–400 pages. By then, development of low-cost multi-track copying machines and small, portable four-track German tape recorders and later four-track compact cassette recorders, made study and the processing of so much material, technologically feasible. Up until then, a reader, if available, would operate on a one-to-one basis, or all materials had to be transposed to Braille.

I was not alone. The history of the blind in education generally has been, to say the least, deeply troubled. Apart from the social stigma and physical exclusion from learning encountered, many believed learning for the blind was 'futile'. Blindness in ancient times and through to the 20th century was filled with few prospects for work, although progressive educators believed that the sense of touch could be used, arguing that ability to see was not central to understanding. It was therefore in 1821 that Frenchman Louis Braille, aged only 15, invented the technique of using a series of raised dots placed within a square so that a code for reading and writing could be developed. Advanced Braille used shorthand contractions for prefixes and suffixes and other abbreviations. Learning this system is not straightforward. Dr Jane Poulson in The Doctor Will Not See You Now, describes learning Braille as 'aggravating' because she constantly lost her place in a page of raised dots.

Largely because of this Braille specialty, education for the blind became channelled through specialised institutions up until recent technology took over.[120]

The Student's Institutional Experience

The participation of students in specialised educational and charitable institutions is, however, mixed. Some argue that they felt they learnt more and were more at ease, but others reported on a harsh and unbending environment. Nevertheless, back in 1975, as I entered the formidable, austere, two storied blue stoned Victoriana building of the RVIB — above its front door an inscription in stained glass read, 'Asylum for the Blind' — I wondered, was this to be like Coleridge's translation of Dante's sign over the entrance to Hell, 'Abandon hope all ye who enter here?' Or was it to be the beginnings of hope and a new life? Sadly, my initial experience was to be negative.

With little welcome or induction, I was shown to a sparsely furnished room without character or homeliness, part of a vast cavernous, echoing second storey wing where it appeared I was all alone. Coming as I had just done, from a warm and welcoming home environment, my little room with its cheap fittings, small table, bed, cupboard and chair was hardly encouraging. My room was serviced by a barren, communal bathroom whose cold concrete floor framed by white institutional tiles, remained interspersed throughout the day by stale, dank puddles of undrained water.

My fears of entering a new world were similar to those expressed by Dr Jane Poulson, who wrote this about commencing rehabilitation in Montreal, Canada: 'I was gripped by panic. Why? Because it was here in this place, in this common room surrounded by people who like me were blind, that I was suddenly hit by the crushing reality of my circumstances. I was like them, truly handicapped ... the blind amongst the blind, I was one of them ... this had suddenly become my world, one I was afraid to enter.'[121]

While I was not totally blind like Jane, my response was similar. As my first day of rehabilitation began, no in-depth assessment of my vision was made to understand what I could or could not see, a methodology I thought necessary in order to understand what my rehabilitation and teaching needs were. It was just presumed that I was blind like others and so I commenced lessons in touch-typing and Braille, then later told to purchase a folding white cane for mobility. In short, it seemed to me that vision impairment for the RVIB extended to universal blindness for everyone, including management.

At this stage, with only minimal central vision loss and having very little peripheral field loss, my mobility was really quite excellent. So, I quickly found the cane of little assistance. In any event, I received no training on how to use the cane, so what was the point of buying it?

I found Braille, although interesting, unhelpful when instead, I could still see enough for organisational purposes using large print and black felt pens. But learning touch-typing turned out to be of invaluable assistance in the short and long term.

With 33 per cent of useable vision in one eye, Janet Shaw from Perth, Western Australia, talks in her book, Beyond the Red Door, about the classic over-reach of a sighted bureaucracy, which, as in my own case, did not comprehend, or perhaps really inquire, what partial vision loss really meant. Janet was placed in a special school for the blind which had a red door to distinguish it from the neighbouring state school.

Janet commented on leaving her mainstream classroom: 'Leaving my friends, my favourite teachers and the school I loved at the end of grade four was devastating for me. I was to enter a foreign world which at times felt like a prison ... why I had been placed at such a school became even more of a puzzle as the strict rules for a prison style institution closed in on me like the slamming of a cell door!'[122]

In talking about his special school experience, Gary Stinchcombe of Victoria, formerly deputy headmaster of RVIB's Burwood School for the Blind, and who experienced childhood retinal detachment, said, 'I boarded from the age of seven onwards. We weren't allowed to put our fingers in our food and a staff member would come with a wooden spoon to whack us across our fingers if we dipped them into our plates. We soon learnt to use our knives and forks, but I guess it was tough love. Maybe it was a good thing!'

However, another special school student, Amelia with albinism, said of her experience at the Burwood School for the Blind 'I hated discipline and what I thought were silly rules. For this reason, I think I was picked on as a trouble maker. One day they just came and said I was a good swimmer and had to go swimming. We had to do thirty laps as a warm up and I had never swum before!' Amelia's bitter experience is supported by Gina, blind from birth with retinopathy of prematurity (ROP), who said, 'I couldn't swim and I was terrified when thrown in the deep end with just a rope around my neck!'

'Sport at the blind school,' said Janet Shaw, 'consisted of jumping and exercising in a small room, not playing net ball soft ball, tunnel ball, or running around an oval. Every day I watched as the children from the sighted school ran around freely, played ball games and sat in little groups on the grass to eat their lunch.'

Bronwyn, while a boarder with the RVIB, said: 'They never taught me to cook a roast dinner. One night Matron came, she like other staff were all dressed up in white uniforms And said, "Bronwyn, you are cooking tea tonight for everyone!" It was roast beef and vegetables. While I had received some cooking instructions I didn't get any instructions or assistance. I just had to do it on my own. I eventually did it, but at the end, I thought others would have to help washing up, but Matron said, "Bronwyn, you are washing up!" and I had to do it all!'

In talking about her West Australian experience, Janet Shaw reported, 'Rules that made no sense, they tried to change me, to break me out of my childhood, to make me someone I clearly wasn't!' To learn Braille, 'Rule one was to use your fingers.' 'No! no! No! You are not to use your eyes!' was the severe remonstration from the teacher when she used her vision. 'I was puzzled, why was I being asked to use my fingers when I could see?'[123]

The De-institutionalisation of Education

As a result of many years of complaints about abuse, inhumane treatment and numerous government inquiries, institutionalisation of people with intellectual and physical disability generally, was regarded as unsuitable and seen as a mechanism of segregation. Institutions were characterised by a regimented culture, limitation of personal possessions and fixed timetables for activities like eating and walking, irrespective of residents' preferences or needs.

De-institutionalisation, the policy supporting closing down of this form of care, was seen as a policy that aimed to reduce long-stay residential facilities and its inequities.

The closure of special schools for the blind and vision impaired took place in line with these general community changes. The solution for children with vision impairment was called 'mainstreaming', meaning closing of special schools and integration of students with special needs into 'mainstream' schools of general public education. This took place during the 1970s in Australia. Janet Shaw wrote, 'Blind students were allowed to mix, use their remaining sight with larger letters, play in the inter-school sport competition. But, the real victory came from just being there!'[124]

As integration took place in Victoria, a Government Special Needs Visiting Teacher Service developed along with a Statewide Vision Resource Centre. Today, there are approximately 4,000 vision impaired students in Australia, most of whom attend mainstream schools.

Some Educational Philosophies

From my own experience and that of other vision impaired students as detailed above, it was thought best that, in moving away from special schools, students with a vision impairment should be held to the same academic, social and behavioural standards as sighted students. Educationalists believe that students:

- who have a vision impairment need to be given the same accessible content to ensure that they acquire what is needed in their subjects
- do not have diminished expectations from their peers
- are prepared for adulthood when they will be judged equally in competitive employment markets
- have the right social skills. Behaviour influences the attitudes of others as a basis for employment, social participation, and community. Sensible socialisation reflects upon students' self-concept and self-esteem.[125]

Reviews of De-institutionalization

To the disappointment of many, mainstreaming did not produce the Golden Goose. Like the de-institutionalisation of similar protective structures in the mental health sector, many ill-prepared and under-resourced people were left to struggle in the general community. In 2015, 'Shut Out', a government report on the effects of de-institutionalisation on the broader disabled community in Australia said, 'The institutions that once housed them [the disabled] may be closed, but the inequity remains. Where once they were physically segregated, many Australians with disabilities now find themselves socially, culturally and politically isolated. They are ignored, invisible and silent. They struggle to be noticed, they struggle to be seen, they struggle to have their voices heard.'[126]

Similar difficulties were noted for students with vision impairment in 2013. A report prepared by Media Access Australia for Blind Citizens Australia (BCA) identified a number of factors inhibiting access to learning for students who are blind and vision impaired. These included:

- Existing structures hindering knowledge sharing between schools, sectors and states
- A lack of opportunities for coordination to prevent duplication of resources
- Copyright issues affecting the availability of texts in alternative formats (Note: This may have been resolved by the 2013 Marrakech Treaty which loosened copyright restrictions on books for the blind.)
- A lack of information to help educators and education departments to adapt to technological change.[127]

As always, individual educators understand the diverse needs and capabilities of disabled children. However, as can be expected, the 'steam roller' of bureaucratic teaching institutions makes it difficult to diversify a syllabus and the method of its delivery. It is difficult for an individual teacher to provide materials in alternative formats. Many young clients reported that accessible technology was unavailable and the delivery was rigid. (See Chapter 15, Schooling Issues.)

The Education Breakout

By the 1970s, with 'mainstreaming' swinging into action, it was emerging technology that provided wonderful solutions. The world of people with vision impairment radically moved into a new era. Information in a digital format and read as audio, displaced Braille as a mainstream form of communication. Until the amazing Artificial Intelligence (AI) voice recognition systems were developed recently, no other change reaped so much benefit so quickly for the vision impaired community.

The introduction of portable reel-to-reel tape recording, then cassette tape recorders in the 1970s as mentioned, provided the first breakthrough in learning. Access to study at all levels dramatically changed. The RVIB and other organisations for the blind developed a Tape Reading Service, which enabled a far wider range of people with vision loss to participate in secondary and tertiary studies than ever before.

The amount of volunteer time to support the Tape Reading Service was immense. To read a large textbook of, say, 500 pages might take up to 144 hours of reading. This was surely a most selfless devotion to this cause. Often readers by mistake, would read over a previously recorded track of say, 90 minutes, only having to read it all again. With over 130 students undertaking several years of study, it can be imagined how much voluntary work was required, but as much as this system worked, it was all swept away by the new digital technology.

Those who did it the hard way include Professor Ron McCallum, who is blind from birth due to oxygen given to him as a premature baby which damaged his retinas. He had numerous volunteer readers, including his mother, reading onto tapes, and also used Braille as notes. Ron completed a law degree and ended up Dean of Law at Sydney University. Professor Laurie McCredie whose sight, hearing and one hand were destroyed by a grenade explosion, studied Law in the 1960s with lots of volunteers reading and became Sub Dean of Monash University Law School in Melbourne. Not being able to type and restricted with Braille, Lawrie dictated his answers to exams. Lawrie's memory was so well developed that his secretary could read to him a five-page Trust Deed — imagine, nothing quite so boring! — and Lawrie could then recite it back –yes, literally word for word![128]

Education drives employment.

A joint Canadian, Australian and New Zealand research study found in 2018, 'A strong link between educational background and full-time employment rates for people with sight loss. In Canada, only 5.5 per cent of people with sight loss who don't have a high school diploma are working full time, versus 35 per cent with a post-secondary degree, compared with Australia, where the statistics were 10.6 per cent versus 28 per cent. In

New Zealand, 15 per cent of people with sight loss who don't have a high school leaving qualification are working full time, versus 42 per cent with a degree.'[129]

A major barrier still remaining for students is the cost of computer hardware and software, although the The National Disability Insurance Scheme (NDIS) will provide some support. The NDIS has been reluctant to pay for everyday technology but will pay for equipment that meets special disability requirements, or configuration, provided it is supported by a technology specialist's report. (Check the NDIS website, https://www.ndis.gov.au, for details, or contact by phone on 1800 800 110 or email enquiries@ndis.gov.au. NDIA, the insurance authority, also produces a 'Price Guide' for the NDIS which should be examined as well.)

However, once a person has a job, the Australian Government's JobAccess program offers financial solutions for the provision of equipment and training.

Some Study Principles

Based upon my experience, some important study principles remain constant. With my own study, I was assisted by a mentor, the late Jim Finn, who became a successful lawyer. By 1976, Jim had only some light perception left following retinal cancer, but his adroit advice on how to study saved me from failure. Jim's advice was:

- Carefully select your topics.
- Ask around to identify and select those lecturers who provide much better structure to their course lectures than others.

- Carefully minimise the amount of reading, and discuss a short list of essential reading with your lecturer.
- Always request additional time for undertaking exams!

The above is great advice still relevant today! Jim also used Braille for his note-taking, typed his exams, developed an excellent memory and successfully conducted his country law practice for many years.

Ross Miller in BCA News[130] argues that it is time to develop a new approach to study as we prepare for a rapidly changing economy and I support these views. Ross says, 'There is a tendency for people with vision impairment to be pushed into traditional roles such as phone and computer contact and support combinations. It is time to develop roles requiring Bachelor of Business, a Masters of Business Administration or similar education standard.' In my experience, becoming manager of an office was infinitely preferable to just administration. Blindness does not inhibit study, learning, developing strategies, research or policy development. However, a person with vision impairment steered into data processing, has little scope for advancement.

We tend not to be aware of, or forget about the achievements of people who were totally blind. As mentioned in Chapter 2, teachers, scientists, mathematicians and medical doctors and lawyers have broken through the blindness barrier, so the scope for greater diversity of career is possible. There will be plenty of disbelievers, though. Ross Miller asks:

- Why not study in one of the STEM areas, Science, Technology, Engineering, Mathematics, economics and business management?

- Why not work from an early age towards these goals like other enthusiastic people in society?
- Why not use skills in organisation, lateral thinking, presentation and strong personal motivation, to move into the larger and often competitive sectors of the workforce?
- Why not be the Manager of Corporate Expansion in a medium sized services business, promoting the company, generating contacts and managing teams and budgets?

Miller goes on to say, 'There are many pathways that can be pursued. The system is there to use, the services are there to support, the research provides lists of future opportunities.'

Broadly speaking, Miller is correct. From my earlier experience as a Chief Executive Officer, the best place to be as a person with vision impairment, is at the top. From a managerial level you can control your work place and work flow. Administration is the least preferred option as it tends to lock an employee in to complex data processing with little scope for promotion — back to the old switchboard employment principle?

However, Ross Miller's educational pathways, 'focus, mentoring and professional training', need to start at an early stage of an educational pathway for those with vision loss. This could be as early as primary school age. As discussed in this book, parents who did not over-protect their children with vision impairment, raised children who naturally understood and believed they could accomplish anything.

As discussed in other chapters, the greatest impediment may be lack of self-belief and confidence, but as noted in Chapter 10, so much of early confidence comes from parents regarding their child as 'normal'. It is therefore critical that parents also understand

and support these educational and work possibilities and not overprotect with smother love or paternalism. It does happen.

An attitude I encountered numerous times was the parent's guilt complex for having a 'blind child'. In a recent case, a mother dominated to the point where her 'child', by now a 35-year-old woman, could not speak for herself. I formed the view that, largely because of the mother's guilt complex and genuine belief that she had to protect her child, this mother took over nearly everything to the point of domination.

If a teaching institution accepts your application to study, it has an obligation to support you. For example, to provide materials in a format accessible to you. Most of these institutions also have a Disability Support Office. Full use of this service should be made in understanding your rights and negotiating a pathway through higher studies.

Regrettably, while all educational institutions have websites on which course materials are located, the sites themselves, especially with some Technical and Further Education (TAFE) colleges and some universities in Australia, are not always accessible for text reading software. One issue is often that course outlines and materials are made available at the last minute. You must let your lecturer know you need more time to access materials and that you need to obtain these essential materials earlier than other students.

You may also need technological support or advocacy support to manage access. In addition, knowledge of your rights under the Commonwealth Disability Discrimination Act 1992 is also important. It is frequently reported that discrimination does still take place, for example, some lecturers display resentment or resistance towards providing extra assistance. Do not underestimate the value of knowing your rights and acting on them; and explore your capacity to access TAFE and university study websites as early as possible. Both Blind Citizens Australia (BCA) and Vision Australia (VA) have advocacy support.

While many students will be using tablets to access information, a computer and touch typing skills are still highly important for handling a large volume of work. With the arrival of voice recognition technology, both Apple Mac computers, Dragon Dictate and, to a newly evolving extent, Microsoft's Narrator, enable you to dictate your assignments and exams. Be sure to carefully refine your dictation skills for conciseness.

Communication and Reading

> 'I don't read to go to sleep, I read to keep awake!'
> Said 33rd US President Harry Truman.

One of the most common complaints from people experiencing vision loss and especially older people with late onset, is 'I can't read!' Their world of books, newspapers, magazines, how to do it instructions, letters, diaries and recipes, all dissolves into a fog of blurredness. What to do?

Reading and the Impact of Neuro-plasticity for Audio Devices

Most sighted people will have developed a strong visual memory and if sight loss occurs they are now required to turn to using aural memory. Many struggle to accept this method believing their memory is inadequate. However, aural neuron pathways get stronger with use. Current knowledge about the brain's neuro-plasticity confirms that our brain is capable of 're-circuiting' neuron pathways with electrical messages.[131] But we have to know and trust this to believe it.

It might surprise those with full sight to know that the vast majority of people with vision impairment, once adjusted to their sight loss, will listen to audio books at twice, sometimes three times the normal speaking rate. This sounds like a super-fast Donald Duck voice, a Duck on Steroids, impossible to understand. But, we get used to it. What this demonstrates is that the brain's neuro pathways have strengthened. We can all do this, and unless there is some cognitive malfunction, this process continues until the day we die!

The Internet and Downloading Books

Most people who have lost their sight later in life struggle with the natural instinct to look at things. The fundamental, ingrained habit of looking is hard to change, which is perhaps one reason why vision loss is so difficult to come to terms with. Many will try to use magnifying glasses or CCTV scanners, or enlarge the text on their computers, but these methods can be frustrating, slow and ineffective compared to the low cost and effectiveness of text-to-speech audio reading devices.

One of the outcomes of this loss is the grief that arises when we can no longer read books. People report, 'It is their touch, smell and sheer practicality which we miss.' It stands to reason that it is also hard for someone to become attached to plastic, hard, impersonal, confusing technology, downloading and 'the cloud' technology. For older people, use of modern gadgets requires a great deal of re-skilling.

Modern technology has had a profound difference in enabling access to information, including books and newspapers, the web, movies and theatre. It is quite accurate and really exciting to say, 'There are no longer any barriers to information access.' Let's look at why.

With audio software such as JAWS, NVDA in computers and Voice Over and Talk Back in smartphones, nearly all text information on the web is accessible. (See Chapter 18, Technology and Working in the Shed.)

For audiobooks, with the worldwide movement to cloud technology and downloading information, the traditional tapes and CDs have almost disappeared. Public libraries still have a range of audio CDs but even these are changing to a single MP3 disk or DVD. You can digitally borrow audiobooks from sites such as BorrowBox, Libby and Overdrive. You can purchase books from Amazon, Audible and other web sites including:

- Library Genesis. ...
- Centsless Books. ...
- Project Gutenberg. ...
- ManyBooks. ...
- Feedbooks. ...
- PDFBooksWorld.
- Open Library.

Most blindness agencies have audio libraries with audiobooks. Book Share is a US E Library with over 600,000 titles. Non-audio books can be downloaded via Amazon, or I books, or Audible, but can be read using smartphones with in-built Voice Over, or Android's Talk Back.

The 2016 Marrakesh Treaty has allowed waiving of copyright restrictions for people with vision impairment and allow access to a greater diversity of materials.

Access to audio-based information includes access to daily and regional newspapers, magazines and podcasts downloaded by way of an app called VA Connect, available free from Google Play or Apple's App Store. However, you need to register to be a member of Vision Australia's library to obtain a password, but this is a free service like other public libraries. You can also get training to use the app if needed. The VA Connect app can be used on all smartphones and tablets. Downloading is also possible via desktop or laptop computer.

Other Devices for Reading

Apart from smartphones and tablets, there are other excellent reading devices available.

About the size of a packet of cigarettes, the VictorReader Stream (available from humanware.com) costs about AU$500. Its advantages are:

- it's very portable size
- its battery life of 16 hours

- its ability to store an entire library of books, depending on the size of the SD card
- wifi for easier downloading (on recent models).

Envoy Connect is a small, solar-powered or rechargeable device capable of carrying 20 books and with a battery life of 30 hours. While simple to use, its speaking rate cannot be increased. It is available from Vision Australia (https://shop.visionaustralia. org/shop).

Audio Description (AD)

A typical response of vision impaired people is, 'I no longer go to the theatre or movies. I can't see what's going on, so there's no point!' Well, if that is how you, your family or other friends think, think again because AD breaks this barrier down. The audio description (AD) service can change your life.

For live and musical theatre, the AD service has volunteers who describe the set, action between dialogue and other unspoken parts. With movies, a professional description is included in the movie (and also on the DVD if you are listening at home). The service is free, but you need to ask your theatre or cinema when 'audio described' shows are on and book this service. At the venue, you will be given a hand set with headphones to listen to the audio description. 'This is an amazing service and it has changed my feelings about going to the movies altogether!' is the typical response on using this service.

Most modern TV's Sony, Phillips and Samsung now have voice activated menus and operations. When purchasing a new TV, make sure this feature is included.

AD is available for Australian TV channels ABC and SBS. To access audio description on relevant programming, televisions and/or set top boxes must have audio description settings enabled. Many devices will require the assistance of a sighted person to adjust these settings in the first place and it is recommended you take the time to set up your device ahead of the program to ensure you have audio description enabled.

To set up audio description you will need to update the audio language setting on your device using your remote control and on-screen menu options, or activate the accessibility features of your equipment. Settings will vary between brands. Both the ABC and SBS websites include instructions for setting up audio description on a large number of tested television models. You can also check your device manual or contact your manufacturer for specific information about your equipment if needed. As an AD program starts, a chime can be heard; or check web sites for AD listed programs.

AD is available in the UK, New Zealand, Canada, Europe and other countries. To get latest AD schedule of AD events, contact Vision Australia on 1800 84 74 66, or email: Michael.Ward@visionaustralia.org.

12

Employment and Discrimination

'Blind eyes can perceive more than an ignorant mind.'

Professor Dr Faisal Khosa

'Last November a large midwestern university was looking for a man to teach public law. Having read my published articles but knowing nothing else about me, the head of the department in question wrote a letter to the University of California inquiring whether I would be available for the position. I replied that I would and accompanied the answer with a considerable collection of supporting material. However, when the department head learned that I was blind, the deal was off although none of the competing applicants had as good a papers showing.'

Professor Dr Jacobus tenBroek, first president of the

US NFB and winner of the Woodrow Wilson Award for outstanding book of the year in political science

The Struggle for Employment

In 1980, when I tentatively ventured into the employment lists, I had to rely on volunteer readers organised by the Royal Victorian Institute for the Blind (RVIB). I could not have survived my first years of work without their support. Later, when office manager, I deployed secretaries to assist, but I had to be careful not to over-use them just to support me.

When I commenced office work in 1981, the introduction of computers and the internet initially only worsened my work scenario because poorly structured websites and hyperlinks were difficult to access with keyboards and, accordingly, mouse users were masters of this universe. By the mid-1990s, my situation began to dramatically change when text-to-speech audio software called JAWS became available.

After being admitted to practise as a barrister and solicitor in the Supreme Court of Victoria, the High Court of Australia and a host of lesser jurisdictions, I was to find out the legal profession had fallen into a period of temporary, but significant recession. During the last two years of university and my year undertaking articled clerkship, I wrote more than 300 unsuccessful job applications to law firms and other businesses. I was to therefore come to terms with a stark reality, that few employers took on articled clerks and even less were amenable to take on someone with vision impairment.

I came to the disheartening conclusion that employers were more receptive to accepting people with other disabilities than poor vision, based on groundless fears of how a person with vision loss could cope. The days where administrative staff were plentiful had long since gone. Practitioners were now required to undertake increasing amounts of administrative tasks and one-on-one support was less likely.

One incident was particularly hurtful. In 1981, I had applied for a position of Tutor at the Royal Melbourne Institute of Technology (RMIT) and by phone, had been offered the job. After visiting the lecturer in charge to discuss my low vision and make sure he understood my differing work requirements, shortly afterwards I received a phone call from him to say the position no longer existed. Despite the feelings of blatant discrimination, there was nothing I could do, no way, based on these verbal exchanges, I could prove discrimination. So angry and smarting with this rejection, I cursed, then carried on, somewhat disillusioned to join a list like hundreds of others in the reject pool.

Of course, like Professor Dr Jacobus tenBroek, I'm not the only person with vision impairment to have faced discrimination: the attitudes of the sighted towards the blind, as Helen Keller said, are the greatest barriers. As with the example of Professor Jacobus tenBroek, adventurer Erik Weihenmayer experienced discrimination when trying to get a job as a dishwasher: 'I hadn't realised that there were doors that would remain locked in front of me,' he writes in his book Touch the Top of the World. 'I didn't get a dishwasher job that year in Cambridge, but I did choke down an important lesson. That people's perceptions of our limitations are more damaging than those limitations themselves. It was the hardest lesson I ever had to swallow.'[132]

The only conspicuous examples of totally blind lawyers

succeeding at the time I completed my studies in 1980, were two blind barristers, Gillespie-Jones from Canberra and Smith from Melbourne, while the dynamic, totally blind Kate McKenzie, worked as a legislative draftsperson with the Victorian Parliament. My mentor, the redoubtable Jim Finn, had attempted to become a barrister, but he too found the going too hard and became a country solicitor. The success rate for lawyers or barristers with vision loss in private practice was low. For the most part they became academics, or were engaged in policy roles for government, where work scope and working conditions were more clearly defined.

In recent times, Darren Fittler of Gilbert Tobin from Sydney and Robert Altmore working with the federal government, demonstrate how totally blind people can succeed in Law. Even the amazing Laurie McCredie, one-time Sub Dean of Monash University's Law School told me how difficult legal practice could be in the 1960s. As an officer in the army he was critically injured in a training accident. Following rehabilitation at St Dunstan's in England — a training school for the blind — and completing a law degree at Melbourne University, he resigned from his law office after overhearing two partners of the firm discussing him one day, saying: 'It's a pity about Lawrie's eyesight, if it weren't for that, he would be made a partner!' Angered by this patent display of bias, Lawrie resigned and took up an academic post at Monash University Law School, wrote law books and proved how blindness was not a barrier.[133]

Research led by the Canadian National Institute for the Blind found that people with sight loss are significantly less likely to be employed full time compared to their sighted counterparts. 'In a survey of blind and partially sighted adults across three countries, results showed Australia had the lowest full-time employment rate at 24 per cent, followed by Canada at 28 per cent, while New Zealand had the highest with only 32 per cent. However, the full-time employment rate among the general public in these countries, in some cases, is nearly double that.'[134]

While employment rates vary among people with disability, those with sensory or speech impairment have the highest labour force participation rate at 56.2 per cent.[135] But for those with vision impairment, according to Blind Citizens Australia (BCA), only 24 per cent of people with vision impairment have full-time work.[136] The CEO of Vision Australia also confirmed (21 March 2019) that 'Less than 30% of people who are blind or have low vision have full time employment'.

In 2018, in referring to all disabilities, the Australian Human Rights Commission stated, 'Australia ranks lowest among OECD countries for the relative income of people with disabilities. Overall employment rates for people with disabilities remain low, with workforce participation at around 54 per cent compared to 83 per cent for people without disabilities. Switzerland appears to have the highest disability employment rate of 69%. People with disability continue to have lower rates of labour force participation.'[137]

Dealing with Discrimination and Disclosure

In most cases middle management has the role of appointing new staff and, of course, they don't have the authority to take risks. What a brave decision it must be to employ a person who is blind! For this reason, and taking into account woeful figures for employment rates of people with vision impairment as mentioned above, an employer who states they are an 'Equal Opportunity Employer' would appear to be offering mere tokenism. Perhaps these employers who seek to hold out this status as a sign of their stature, should have to account for and report their employment rates of disabled people.

Even Vision Australia, the leading provider of services for the blind and vision impaired, has seen its employment rate for people with vision impairment fall from 18.5 per cent in 2009, to less than 14 per cent in 2019. In 2021, only one senior second-tier manager with significant vision loss remained.

It is the decision makers of organisations who need to understand that the working capacities of vision impaired people are excellent and it is they, the decision makers, who must clear this blockage within their organisations. On important factors in selecting prospective employees, Sandra Budd, Blind Foundation of New Zealand's Chief Executive states, 'We see a great opportunity in supporting employers to make changes that result in more inclusive workplaces for people with sight loss. This is the same at the government level — systemic change in accessibility and inclusion will help to move us forward.'[138]

The joint Canadian, Australian and New Zealand blindness organisations 2018 research referred to earlier, also points to the 'need for a shift in employer attitudes and business practices to help make workplaces more accessible for people who are blind or partially sighted. The survey showed 43 per cent of Australian respondents identified their workplace's inaccessibility as a barrier compared to 58 per cent of Canadians and New Zealanders. Additionally, more than 60 per cent of respondents in all three countries believe employer attitudes are one of the main barriers to full-time employment –half reporting feeling they had not been hired because of their sight loss.'[139]

Disclosure

A dilemma facing most people with vision impairment is, how much should I tell my employer about my vision loss and when? That is, should a person with vision loss declare their disability in their job application and, if they were to get one, reveal this in their interview? Naturally, there are some with total vision loss and those who need a white cane or dog guide for mobility, who really have no option. However, the greater percentage of people with vision loss who have varying degrees of sight, face a difficult choice. The general view is, do not declare sight loss unless you really have to! However, this stance raises a difficult ethical dilemma: should your disability be disclosed? On the other hand, why should employers who continue to demonstrate undisclosed prejudice and not employ those with vision disability, also not disclose their bias and remain protected by not having to reveal reasons for their decision? Naturally they fear discrimination claims, but this imbalance does seem a little unfair. Perhaps only arbitrary quotas, or transparent reporting of the numbers of disabled people employed by organisations, or government intervention, can fix this situation.

One example of how tough it is to gain employment is illustrated by my own experience. Between 1979 and 1980, I made over 300 job applications. In most I included a carefully worded paragraph stating that, 'All of my achievements have been attained despite having a vision impairment.' I did not get a single interview. When

I left out this paragraph from some applications, I was invited for an interview about 50 per cent of the time.

The question is, then, how much should be disclosed about your disability? While employers remain unaccountable, the imbalance remains.

The often intense emotional struggles of people with vision loss and, of course, people with disability generally, should surely be taken into account when determining employment guidelines. Unless disability is more patently welcomed and understood, barriers brought about through ignorance and doubt will remain.

As noted in the introduction to this book, 75 per cent of Australians surveyed had very little social contact with disabled people. We can hardly expect this to suddenly change when employment takes place.

US commentator Barbara Pierce states, 'People with vision impairment should not expect concessions.' From my own experience, this is basically correct, we still have to compete in an open market-place and this requires adequate education and preparation. But, the playing field is not a level one, so what then is going to be the equaliser? Given the prejudice and discrimination I have already mentioned, Government can assist by creating clearer and stronger rules.

Obtaining Redress

From another perspective, appeals on discrimination under Australia's Disability Discrimination Act 1992 (Commonwealth) are rarely meaningful and do not appear to change day-to-day practice.

Even within the Australian Government Public Service itself, the percentage of people with disability employed is believed to have fallen from approximately 6.5% to 2.9% over the past 10 years.[140] With numbers of employees in the Australian Public Service falling, employment outlook appears limited.

While the following outcomes refer primarily to the disability sector generally and no specific data is available for people who are blind or who have vision loss, these results appear disheartening. The Australian Department of Social Services states in a report in 2014 called Shut Out,[141] 'People with disabilities believe little progress has been made in challenging prevailing attitudes towards disability. Submissions suggested that there are still widespread misconceptions and stereotypes informing the attitudes and behaviour of service providers, businesses, community groups, governments and individuals.'

As a result, Shut Out reports that 'discrimination is a feature of daily life for many people with disabilities and their families. More than 39 per cent of submissions identified discrimination and rights as a vital issue, with one submission noting, virtually every Australian with a disability encounters human rights violations at some point in their lives and very many experience it every day of their lives.'

Submissions to the Victorian Parliament's Social Inclusion and Victorians with Disabilities inquiry in 2014, also made it clear that, 'One important reason discrimination had become so systematic and entrenched was the lack of redress.' Other submissions noted that, 'legislation protecting the rights of people with disabilities is inconsistent across jurisdictions, and there is a remarkable lack of monitoring and enforcement of standards and no effective independent complaints process.'

A number of submissions argued that the process to lodge a complaint under the Disability Discrimination Act 1992 (Commonwealth) is onerous and relies too heavily on individuals being prepared and able to take part in lengthy and costly legal proceedings.[142]

Two national inquiries by the Law Reform Commission and the Human Rights Commission into the issue of access to justice for people with disability identified significant barriers. The 2012 Civil Society Report to the United Nations Committee on the Rights of Persons with Disabilities (Civil Society Report) noted that people with disability experience significant barriers in participating in Australian legal systems 'with many finding access to justice too difficult, hostile or ineffectual'.

A further consideration is that the significant personal stress and financial cost involved in making a complaint prevents many from taking their concerns forward.

There is also a likelihood of such complainants becoming stigmatised as 'trouble makers'. Even within the workplace, complaints or criticism from people with disabilities are hosed down in order to maintain a positive public profile.

Reforms in this area are therefore required.

Some Principles of Employment

With employment, people with vision impairment need to observe four broad principles:

1. If you are already employed and in a role that depends on good eyesight, for example, driving, do not resign just because your eyesight is failing and you think you can no longer carry on. Once out of employment it is very, very difficult to get back in. Have the role assessed by Workplace Assessment Teams, negotiate how your role could be modified and what technological changes can be made, undertake re-skilling in technology as required and use the Australian Government's JobAccess program to support any workplace modifications. There is, after all, a broad recognition within government policy (at least in theory!) that it is better to keep people in employment than have them turn to social welfare.

2. Think carefully about how you can present your vision disability to your workplace. Carefully outline to your team when you need assistance and what kind of assistance is needed. Try to avoid the impression that you are always in need of assistance. This requires you to be up to date with current technology.

3. As approximately 75 per cent of jobs are found by networking (some say the figure is 95 per cent) — plan your work ambition and ascertain how your networks can assist. This is, of course, very difficult for those just entering the workforce, or those with vision impairment whose families do not have access or contacts to employment; nevertheless, it's important to consider what networks are out there. Employment agencies also need to have a 'spotter' employed who can identify suitable roles and negotiate with employers for a fair hearing, an approach that tends to offset barriers referred to above. It is also critical for employment agencies

to understand what vision loss means and that its impact upon each individual is different.

4. Use your non-working time to fully re-skill yourself with your professional, technological, interview and application skills. Take full advantage of in-house training and request workplace modifications to remain effective. Discuss your technology and training needs with specialists.

Unless an employment agency has specific knowledge of disability, they may say they can assist you but only to have you on their 'books'. This again highlights the sometimes abysmal lack of understanding by governments and people with full sight; or perhaps what we're dealing with here is just plain 'dumbness'. But, fear and ignorance held by people with full sight does exist as a barrier and agencies really do need to know what extent of useable sight a client has in order to find appropriate work.

Future Employment Prospects

Writing for BCA News,[143] Ross Miller looked at the future of work and emphasizes how improvements in technology will have repercussions for the workforce in general, not just those with vision loss. The workforce generally is adopting high-tech and artificial intelligence and the high dependence of vision impaired workers on technology will not give them much advantage. he points to how some vocational agents are referring people with vision impairment into job areas such as 'switchboard, customer service and production or reception roles which are mostly disappearing.'

One essential problem of agencies is that they have little need to be creative or take risks in 'considering previously discounted pathways'.

If the UK survey, referred to above, is any indicator, then we are dealing with a fundamental block when it comes to sighted people accepting that blind people can hold down a job. Miller suggests that people with vision impairment, in considering their education, need to think about 'broader options such as non-traditional commerce and industry sectors', preferably taking back control through entrepreneurial approaches. There is also a danger that those with disability are provided with the 'dignity of employment, but then hidden away and forgotten', Miller says.

To quote Barbara Pierce from the US again,[144] 'The problem of finding and keeping a good job is many-faceted, but there is a social component to it. One must have an accurate notion of what is required by an employer. One must meet or preferably exceed those requirements. This is difficult if parents, teachers, and fellow students have been making allowances because of one's visual impairment. Charity will not and should not be part of the equation. We must demonstrate a willingness to work as hard and as competitively as possible. Co-workers often assume they will have to look out for and make allowances for a vision impaired worker', but this can be avoided.

Support in Gaining Employment

The employment services of blindness agencies in Australia have limited geographic coverage. Their links with other agencies that don't necessarily understand vision loss are not helpful. However, blind agency support from Vision Australia offers:

- preparation of resumes
- skills in job application techniques
- training in technology and workplace modifications with follow-up training
- how to respond to Key Performance Indicators (KPIs) — sometimes called Key Performance Criteria — usually a 'must' to complete
- developing successful interview skills
- workplace assessment for your job
- Braille training
- at Kensington, Victoria, a Jobseekers' Club — speakers selected from special areas or from how other people with vision impairment succeeded
- computer training, which includes JAWS, magnification, zoom or Windows Magic, typing speed accuracy, managing emails, using Outlook with calendar and Excel spreadsheets. With low vision, how to use CCTV in filling in forms
- mobility and your personal presentation.

With the introduction in Australia of the National Disability Insurance Scheme (NDIS), support may now be available for equipment that is 'reasonable and necessary, is specific for vision loss and not funded elsewhere'. Check with your Agency or on line.

13

Teenagers, Men, and Issues of Vision Loss and Socialisation

'Just because you are blind, and unable to see my beauty doesn't mean it does not exist.'
Margaret Cho, actor, comedian, singer and song writer

'If you truly want to be respected by people you love, you must prove to them that you can survive without them.'
Michael Bassey Johnson, The Infinity Sign

Teenagers: Dealing with Social Pressures and Self-care

Over 14 years, I found conducting discussion groups for teenagers, and understanding their educational and self-care needs, to be most difficult of all groups. I recall the story of Rose, a girl of 14 years living in rural New South Wales. With RP, Rose began to present complex learning and relationship behaviours. Unable to see clearly, she refused to use adaptive technology in the schoolroom because 'I don't want to look different to the others!' Her response to her mother's deep concern was one of avoidance. 'I want to leave school, get a job and go out working with Dad!' she said. When I attempted to make further contact, she declined participation in a teenagers' group.

It appears to me that, not unsurprisingly, for many teenagers still struggling to establish an identity, avoidance of vision issues was the preferred option. Accordingly, I summarise some key factors.

Rose's response was typical. Sadly, many teenagers refused to talk about their sight loss. Often they remain in their room — one boy who suffered intense glare, to the despair of his mother, only came out in the evenings, or worked all night on his technology — a response that obviously distresses parents. While logic might say that teenagers might prefer sophisticated technology, the reality of peer-group pressure is that teenagers like Rose say they do not like having some special reading device or computer on their desk when their classmates do not.

As teenagers, with or without sight, social pressures and social conformity with mates are primary factors. US social commentator Barbara Pierce states it clearly for girls,[145] 'As blind girls approach adolescence, the social problems they face multiply and become more complex. A solid foundation of social skills established in childhood becomes ever more important for a child's socialisation and learning. The girl who cannot flip through clothing catalogues, observe what girls her age are wearing, or take note of clothing in the stores is at a disadvantage in dressing. Flattering and up-to-date hair styles, appropriate and skilfully applied make-up and recognition of attractive body contours can be equally mysterious to a young blind girl.'

Barbara goes on to say, 'If they are part of the picture, friends can be more useful here than adults, but lack of support could widen the gap in friendships. Blind girls must learn the importance of the information they are lacking, and then the deficit must be made up. They must then learn to assume the responsibility for gathering such information for themselves in the future.'

Some Tips for Girls

I recommend the guide to self-care and grooming by Young Blind Citizens Australia (YBCA), 'Blind Living: Hair, Beauty and Fashion'.[146]

The YBCA guide says, 'Perhaps you did spend ages in front of the mirror, or looking at clothes, becoming exasperated over trying to work out what suited you, how to apply makeup without looking like the queen of smudge, or trying to fix your hair so you didn't look like Cousin It.'

Says Lauren Hayes, President of YBCA. She says, 'As a person who is totally blind, I've certainly found the world of hair, beauty and fashion to be a complicated and confusing place, as have many other blind and vision impaired people I know.'

The Experience of Boys

Many teenage boys who I approached to join discussion groups, flatly refused, or if initially agreeable, failed to attend. As for their reasons, they thought no one could understand their situation, or felt socially awkward, or did not wish to associate with other 'blind' people. In some other instances, parents became overprotective, to such an extent that a boy's refusal was an attempt to be independent. The teenage boys I met appeared to have few friends from school, did not participate in sport, felt they looked 'stupid with thick glasses or sunglasses', or were so limited by their vision they could not participate in the usual games and sport, independently go out, or drive and follow the typical social life enjoyed by others.

I found teenagers with vision loss of both sexes largely dominated by an overwhelming lack of confidence, much more than the ordinary teenager.

Blind mountaineer, writer and adventurer, Erik Weihenmayer when in his early teens, refused to accept his vision loss. Erik tells of when his school driver said to him one day, 'Erik, you may not want to be blind, but you are. The answer isn't always to fight, let people in. Let them help you for a while, you might just learn to catch [a ball] again.' Erik said, 'Independence didn't come in leaping strides, but in tiny successes, almost imperceptible. It came with the discovery that I could match my socks by using safety pins ... in the pride of obtaining an "A" paper written on my speech adapted computer and in the confidence that in knowing my surroundings by the clues I felt through the end of a white cane. Although small, they gave me the courage to dream a little bigger.'[147]

Dating Generally

The teen years are difficult for everyone, and are so much harder for those with vision impairment. To quote again Barbara Pierce, who herself is vision impaired, 'There are certainly some exceptions, but few blind teens have much of a dating life during high school. For the most part sighted teens are so insecure themselves that they do not dare associate romantically with anyone as demonstrably different as a blind person. What is a teen to do during these desert years of "just friendship" with the opposite sex? The short answer is, endure them and gain as much experience as possible!'

Based upon a series of discussions with vision impaired clients, Facilitator Sarah Taylor set out her 'top 5 dating tips' in an article for Vision Australia Community News.[148]

1. Confidence is the elusive quality which, as one could say, is the curse of disability. It's important to have orientation and mobility and occupational therapy skills at a high level. This helps to offset the power-imbalance in relationships where the sighted person becomes your care giver.
2. Apps and online dating. Most dating sites are accessible; however, photos can often be an issue for people. If this is the case have a trusted friend take a photo. Talk to them about what you would like your photo to say about you. It's all about articulating what you want. There are also apps like AIRA that can assist you.
3. Meeting people out and about. Joining special interest groups will assist you to build your confidence. You might not meet the love of your life, but you might meet someone who

knows Mr or Mrs Wonderful. If you're out socially, get a wing-man or wing-woman so they can pick out some potential dates (just make sure they pick out someone you would like and not just someone they would go for).

4. Disclosure. Some people put their disability right out there and other people will wait. Whatever your decision, your blindness or low vision will come up at some point, so be prepared to answer questions. However, keep it brief and focus on the positives and what you can do. For example, maybe you like travel and judo. You do not have to apologise for being blind, for example if your Dog Guide starts grumbling or chewing the furniture.

5. Prepare for the date. Where possible choose the venue yourself. Make it somewhere familiar or research online. Look at the menu, what the opening hours are and public transport options. Don't get your date to pick you up (unless you already know them).

Sarah has a final comment: I would say 'have fun' but anyone who's ever dated knows that this is virtually impossible. So be nice to yourself.

In his book Touch the Top of the World, Erik Weihenmayer has this to say about blindness and boy/girl relationships: 'Some think that people who are blind don't care about looks, that we are above assessing desirability through surface beauty ... in fact I take offense at those who would assume that just because I am blind, I am supposed to be asexual. Blindness has little to do with the virtue or villainy of one's character. My shallowness comes from the voluptuous hum of a sexy voice, the electrifying grasp of a smooth supple hand. It is embarrassing the desperate lengths

I have gone to learn what a woman looks like, while trying to keep alive, her angelic impression of me.'[149]

Men's Issues

Why this section on men and not women? In discussing men's issues, some of my half-forgotten memory surfaced as to how I had initially responded to my diagnosis of having an incurable eye disease. At that time, I was heavily involved in my local Show Committee and with Jaycees. I resigned from these organisations and could not bring myself to even mention, 'I'm going blind!' I couldn't speak about it as I was paralysed by shame and embarrassment, so I quietly withdrew without explanation. I felt it was easier to pull back than face the unspeakable.

I was also to observe, that over the 14 years of conducting group discussions, the majority (approximately 70 per cent) of participants were women, their numbers confirming their greater preparedness to discuss emotional and social issues. Generally speaking, men's issues about blindness and vision loss did not surface to the same degree in my groups. It seems therefore appropriate that some space is made for men's issues.

The physiological impact of vision loss for men need not be any less or greater than for women, but because of established work and family roles, and differences in social skills, the impact for men and their families can be worse. Statistically, in Australia, more men remain principal breadwinners, while salaries for men are usually higher on average than for women. The full-time total remuneration gender pay gap based on Workplace Gender Equality Agency (WGEA) data, is 20.8 per cent, meaning men working full-time earn nearly $25,679 a year more than women working full-time.[150] While the gender pay gap has narrowed, little has changed in the past decade.[151] In the UK, 74 per cent of large and medium-sized companies pay men more than women.[152]

Despite their current economic advantage to women, from particulars provided in discussion groups, the social/economic effect of vision loss for men is harder for them to come to terms with than it is for women, largely because of the employment role models mentioned above.

In special interest men's groups, issues arising as a result of vision loss include:

- a breakdown in relationships with wives and families brought about by loss of income and role changes plus the man's inability or unwillingness to discuss emotions
- a high degree of relationship separation, up to 50 per cent, including where partners left the relationship because of relationship issues, anger and some destructive behaviours attributed to vision loss
- finding that asking for help in the community was difficult because it was embarrassing to explain sight loss in a context where the successful male was breadwinner
- not being able to drive down to the local hotel or sports club to mix with friends, play sport, keep in touch with friendship groups and carry on with a traditional role where 'Dad always drove.
- Asking for help, can you drive me.'

Other common issues identified by group participants include:

- loss of work colleagues and friends
- an inability to use technology (many males in the age range of 40–65 years and in trades, mechanical or factory roles were not necessarily computer fluent)
- having to deal with sighted people's apparently intrusive responses to their sight loss, where explanations were awkward and the man was stoically reluctant to admit disability
- the dismissive attitudes of professionals, including doctors, where no treatment or cure was possible
- the impact on self-esteem: seeing loss of work and a salary as failure
- not using ID badges or white canes out of pride and as a result bumping into others when walking in the street, or not recognizing them
- not knowing what adaptive equipment for jobs existed and lacking capability to use it.

In explaining men's strong feelings arising from loss of work, an American survey found that men face a lot of pressure to support their family financially (76 per cent) and to be successful in their job or career (68 per cent). A much smaller share say women face similar pressure in these areas. At the same time, 75 per cent or more say women face a lot of pressure to be an involved parent and be physically attractive (71 per cent).[153]

Role Changes

In my discussion groups, most men believed loss of employment was perhaps their greatest setback. Apart from clear difficulties regaining employment once you have vision impairment, research by the Australian Human Rights Commission in 2018 confirms that 30 per cent of organisations surveyed were 'reluctant or unwilling to hire anyone over the age of 50'. So, what chance if you are disabled?

What about hobbies? Working in the shed, machinery maintenance, motor rallies, hunting, home maintenance and so on are further areas identified in group discussions which cause frustrations and feelings of low self-esteem after vision loss. These negative feelings can be overcome, of course, usually by realising re-skilling and re-training can identify different ways of doing tasks. Relying upon friends for support makes a difference too.

To deal with these complex topics, I usually invited totally blind men as motivational speakers. In this way I confirmed it was possible for people with vision impairment to carry out motor and car repairs and maintenance, home repairs and maintenance, lawnmowing and gardening, ballroom dancing, electrical work, a vast range of hobbies and sports, woodwork and welding. In fact, there were very few activities which could not be carried out by a person with total blindness. For example, totally blind men and women maintain active lives with activities such as golf, archery, lawn and ten-pin bowls, tennis, sailing, fishing, cricket, scuba diving, sky diving, bushwalking, running marathons and trekking, indoor carpet bowls and Swish (similar to ping pong). Even car driving is possible — usually once a year at events organised with a driving instructor and a car adapted for dual control.

One alpha sports performer, Erik Weihenmayer, who climbed Mount Everest, said of mountain climbing, 'I was realising that the beauty of climbing was joining the incongruent parts [of the rock] to link the cracks, grooves, balls, nubbins, knobs, ledges, and pockets and convert it all into a roadmap etched in my mind. So, by thrashing, groping and bloodying the rock, I worked my way up the face and despite the difficulty, had powered my body up the piece of rock which seemed impossibly foreign to a horizontal world. ... Blindness I thought was a damned nuisance forcing me to climb in a different way to most, but it hadn't stopped me from doing it, or even loving it.'[154]

Mountaineering of course, is not for everyone. However, one major rule of the high achievers is that participation is usually supported by a friend, team or club. For example, Weihenmayer relied upon a team of fellow mountaineers, while world champion cyclist Janet Shaw rode tandem. Blind Sports organisations conduct sport and recreational activities, regularly offering running partners. Totally blind people overcame issues when going fishing by getting a mate to drive and take them to the fishing spot, or club house, help with boat fit-out and launching, handling and baiting fishing lines, and so on. Many keen fishermen like totally blind Gary Stinchcombe, says he can quite easily set up and attach fish hooks, 'It's just a matter of practice!'

When vision loss is recent, it is hard to believe such outcomes are possible, but as discussed throughout this book, it is all about attitude; if you want to do something, you can.

For those men interested in competitive sport, blind and

vision impaired athletes and teams can participate in national championships which can also lead onto the Paralympics. These sports include athletics, cricket, equestrian events, goalball, golf, judo, karate, lawn bowls, powerlifting, rowing, sailing, swimming, tandem cycling, tenpin bowling, water skiing, wrestling and winter sports.

The inability to drive has a particularly big impact on men, affecting their roles in everyday activities such as travel to work, shopping and driving children to school or sporting activities. These roles taken for granted, make adjustment difficult when attributed to a 'personal defect' such as vision loss. It is not easy to change and take up another option like public transport. Public transport is also not always a realistic option in remote or rural areas. Friends might be able to help out, but sometimes home relocation needs to be considered.

Dating For Men

A common area identified in discussions that continues to deeply concern men with vision loss was their inability to engage in early eye contact with women. Much traditional male–female social and sensual contact relies upon early facial recognition and eye contact where sexual desire is often aroused. There is no simple answer to this primordial impulse, and, while many say relationships do not depend upon these methods anyway, there is no simple alternative here. As already mentioned, Blind mountaineer Erik Weihenmayer, writes that many people think that because you are blind you are asexual; this is of course nonsense and both blind men and women share the same sexuality and sexual orientation as sighted people. He trained his friends to give certain signals by way of handshakes to indicate the attractiveness of women as they approached to speak to his dog 'Wizard'.

However, many men with vision impairment felt overwhelmed by inadequacy, and conclude that, 'No woman would be interested in a blind man!' or 'What's the point of going out if I can't see?' These are genuine and serious male attitudes, but nevertheless, due recognition must also be given to how vision impaired females respond in this world of sexual attraction as noted earlier. Solutions do exist and I will mention a few, which can apply to both sexes. (See also Dating, above.)

- Go out with existing male or female friends, or mixed couple friendship groups who do know about and understand your sight loss and can act as 'spotters' for you. Vision impairment gives you no special consideration, you are still required to present yourself as an attractive person.
- Use your existing friendship group to find dates and make introductions for you through non-threatening events such as social nights, dinner parties etc.
- Join mixed sex social clubs such as Probus and become involved in sub-committees, making sure your organisational skills are competent — i.e., you are technologically skilled. Don't become a 'wall flower hoping for sympathy'.
- Join sporting clubs for people with sight loss, such as blind golf; anything is possible.

Consider internet dating sites as a last resort because, while long-distance relationships are possible, for those with money there is danger of financial exploitation. The vulnerability of those on the rebound from an earlier failed relationship is well known. If a genuine contact is made where your vision loss is understood and not exploited, you will still need to be extra careful your partner accepts disability. Going out for the first date, driving, and managing unfamiliar surroundings still presents the usual problems.

When entering into a relationship, as earlier discussed, I strongly recommended that you do not use the word 'blind' if you are partially sighted; instead, use less confronting terms such as 'poor eyesight' or 'bad eyesight'. It is easy to offset your feelings of inadequacy and self-pity by saying 'I'm blind,' just because you cannot see well and you might feel despondent, or self-pitying, but do so only tips you into a pit of increasing negativity. This can be an inadvertent step too far.

Many blind people I've met say that joining a group or organisation where other people with blindness or vision impairment participate is where the strongest relationships and friendships have occurred.

Self-care

Many of the self-care tips applying to women, also naturally apply to men. Good dress sense is important, not allowing clothes to become mis-matched or stained. Personal hygiene is as relevant for men as girls. It is helpful to have a friend or family member you can tolerate, to advise you on dress codes and presentation. Some now use the AIRA or be my eyes apps which uses professionally trained people to act as your 'sighted guide' in describing things for you.

Some skills include:

- keeping up appearance and fashion with hair styles, clothes and recreation
- developing blindness mobility skills and the confidence, which comes from knowing that you can cope in any situation (and this includes being comfortable asking for help)
- asking friends to help and that they understand the sighted guide techniques for going out, reading menus, identifying friends, advising on how others look, taking you to the toilet, driving you out as 'just normal', etc.
- keeping in touch with news, current events and reading with audiobooks means you will be up to date with normal social chat
- joining Telelink groups, or computer based phone technology groups, which include sporting tip competitions and social groups. (Telelink is a 'social and recreational' program conducted by Vision Australia where participants are dialled in free of charge. Topics range from book discussions to sport and crossword contests.)
- listening, really listening, to others who care, and respond with care and tact.

In purchasing clothes, don't pretend to see price tickets or sizes which automatically place you on the back foot. Instead, either go to the shop assistant and ask for help with your selection (keeping in mind that some assistants might over-promote an item) or use a family member or friend to help. If you use the internet, you could send a photo of an item you're interested in to a friend to advise on its suitability before purchasing.

One issue frequently raised by men who experience sudden and total sight loss is, 'How do I not make a mess when standing to urinate at a toilet bowl? (Public urinals do not present such difficulties, only finding out where they are presents problems, although an app called 'find the loo,' may help.) A matter that often came up in my groups was one of considerable embarrassment to men who lost their sight later in life. While some men with blindness choose to sit on the toilet, others prefer to stand because it makes them feel like 'a normal male'. What you need to do is, after making sure you are facing a standard domestic toilet, check the seat is lifted, ensure you can just feel the beginning of the bowl's oval shape between your knees and make sure you are 'squared' to face the cistern. Then, if there is a wall behind the cistern, place your forearm on the wall, then lean over placing your head on your arm. Given average male physiology, and your member is flaccid, urine should safely reach the water in the bowl.

Relax

The great message of relationships is 'friendship'. That is, people will like you for who you are, provided you present a pleasant personality. Often, men and women with vision loss become too negative, and no one likes a complainer. Humour, of course, is always great in developing friendships for men and women. After all, why do we want to congregate in friendship groups? It's all about fellowship; this does not depend upon sight.

Personal Care, Tips for Women and Men

Personal care and using make-up can be a cause of much frustration. It is hard to change from using your vision to trusting your touch. Joanne, a peer from New South Wales, said that despite losing sight from MD, she found that touch allowed her to accurately apply make-up.

Tips for Women

- Use smartphone apps to identify products and read instructions. (See Chapter 18, for more details.)
- Use a hair band to keep hair off your face.
- Use fingers to apply and use wet hand washer to clean.
- Use moisturiser to soften before applying make-up.
- Buy tinted moisturiser.
- Store creams in the fridge to make them stiffer.
- Use an occupational therapist to assist and re-skill, or a reliable friend.
- Use one pump of a dispenser in your hand for one side of the face and again for other side.
- Ask friends to help.

Based on her own experience, Joanne has given these additional tips:

- General: go slowly and practise feeling the key features of your face. You can feel cheekbones, edges of lips, nose etc. After practice, you use muscle memory when you feel your face; you don't have to see.

- With limited sight, consider changing lighting and using a friend to assist.
- Apply lipstick and mascara using a tube; for foundation, apply mineral powder lightly — tap a little bit into the lid and apply with brush.
- Blushes: Joanne tends not to use them as these can be hard to regulate colour.
- Mascara: place it on tips of eyelashes.
- Eye liner: use soft pencil.
- Eye shadow: use finger to lightly soften.
- Eyebrows: use a product with beeswax.

Tips for Men

- Shaving: it's about breaking the habit of looking in a mirror. Instead, use touch to feel what you've missed, where shaving cream is. Best to use an electric razor — it's easier.
- Identify spots like moles; place your finger upon them and shave around them.
- Brushing hair, or needing haircut: you can use touch to feel.
- Have a clear system for maintaining personal hygiene and yes, always ask if your clothes are neat and clean. It's hard at first, but you get used to it.

Tips for both Men and Women

- Wash clothes frequently rather than re-wearing them.
- Keep your shoes in their shoe boxes, have a routine and system for cleaning them or use a clip or bag to keep them together.

- Use organisation gadgets like Pen Friend to read labels you can create for storage items.
- Use colour detector apps for matching colours. The free app, seeing AI, has a colour recognition feature.
- For socks, either use a socks peg, safety pins or bag to keep them together; otherwise, use only one colour — e.g. black.

(14)

Parenting

'Trust yourself. You know more than you think you do.'

Doctor Benjamin Spock

'Parents can only give good advice or put them on the right paths, but the final forming of a person's character lies in their own hands.'

Anne Frank

'The thing about parenting rules is there aren't any. That's what makes it so difficult.'

Ewan McGregor, actor

Overview

Once again, the basis for writing this Chapter was the many hundreds of issues raised when I conducted discussion groups for parents. Every group exposed a desperate need for information on how to be a parent and what are practical tips which make it all possible. Again, the great joy of conducting groups highlighted the fact that just sharing experiences and normalizing this role, was always helpful.

In considering services and supports for parents and children with vision impairment, the wellbeing of parents and the role of the teaching profession can be complex. Firstly, are we dealing with sighted, totally blind or partially sighted parents and children? Or sighted parents with children who have vision impairment? Or parents with vision impairment and fully sighted children? For how long has the disability existed and what are its causes? Are parents dealing with their own issues of coping with vision loss, grief, and emotions of fear or inadequacy? For children, are there issues of identity, acceptance, confidence and skills development? For children with vision loss, positive responses can be easily overshadowed by indeterminate emotional issues, fears, concerns with complex educational issues, bullying and poor handling of children in the school and play environment.

It is important to know there are many successful parents and children with vision loss who, in drawing upon their family values, practical skills and emotional strengths, provide a key resource. Support from dedicated education professionals also plays a critical role. I have listed below typical schooling issues or topics likely to be encountered when vision impairment exists:

- the level of acceptance at home and in the school
- concerns about future careers
- is sight loss stable or deteriorating?

- financial concerns
- required family or career role changes
- access to housing, transport and community services.

As can be seen, the issues are deep-seated, multitudinous and multi-layered.

Some Difficulties

It is a sad fact confirmed by the many personal accounts conveyed in discussion groups, that both children and parents with vision impairment often experience discrimination from the school itself. Teachers who don't understand the impact of vision loss, bullying from other children or avoidance from other parents are among the things that occur. However, we should not set out to blame teachers.

If you are prepared for these issues, then the experience will not be so hurtful.

As Graeme Innes, a totally blind parent says, 'Blindness is of course difficult, but don't be judgemental on yourself. Self-belief and self-esteem come from within. I had a friend who said, 'It's amazing you had kids!' How judgemental is that?'[155]

As earlier discussed, keys to success are accepting your disability and gaining confidence by recognising you can actually do things differently to the way you did them before. Concerns about the future, which we all hold, are made worse by fears of possible future total vision loss. Not knowing that there are solutions is part of a picture exacerbated when children come into the picture.

In a paper on the experiences of parenting with vision

impairment, Rosenblum et al., found that parents' concerns included, 'Expressing concerns about raising children, including protecting their children's safety along with extra time needed to accommodate their own disability and transportation needs, also reported experiencing negative reactions from other people.'[156]

In a number of discussion groups on parenting which I conducted, mothers reported strategies to deal with negative attitudes, such as:

- confiding in other parents
- forming local support groups and joining school committees
- exercising patience in educating other people
- ignoring the negative messages, and learning to laugh about them.

Some Attitudes Worth Considering

Heidi, a totally blind woman in Victoria with four children, provides some extraordinary insights into coping. She says, like our blind parachutist and horse rider earlier referred to, 'it's mostly common sense and determination which gets you there'.[157]

Heidi's view is, 'You struggle every day, missing out on so much going on around you. Understanding this is part of your acceptance journey, your transition can take years. A great reality check is accepting "this is who I am!" It is important to understand that people around you also have grief. Everyone has bad bits and there is nothing miraculous here. If you put values upon your experience, for example, asking is it good or bad? Then this creates expectations you may not meet. Ultimately, be yourself, there is no right or wrong way. Essentially to attain peace within yourself is what is important!'[158]

Family counsellors report, 'Parenting is a daunting undertaking for any individual, but it may be even more daunting for individuals with vision impairments as they think about how to accomplish everyday tasks, such as diapering and transporting children.'[159]

In reflecting upon attitudes to be adopted by those with vision loss, Heidi reported, 'A mother has in-built gut instinct, trust this and give yourself a break! Ask yourself, is this real? Or a perception? Child raising for everyone is a time of transition, you can't stop it. There is of course, the perennial issue of blaming your blindness. Remember, it is not always vision which is the cause, issues of parenting still apply.' As a parent, you are time poor. When operating as a vision impaired person, your mind is busy, if not frantic. You have to remember so much and use adaptive equipment to assist you, for example personal organisers such as audio gadgets. (See Chapter 18, Technology and Working in the Shed.)

As Jenny with diabetic retinopathy in another discussion group said, 'Give yourself time to adjust. Above all, don't feel that you are on show and that you have to be a super parent. Really, just be a parent, your child doesn't see this dilemma. They react to love and nurture which is hard to provide when you are up-tight, stressed or angry!'

Here is some general advice for vision impaired parents.

Managing Young Children

Heidi walks her sighted children to school each day. This presents challenges, of course.

I asked her, 'What did she do when her children became sick at school or it was raining?' Heidi said, 'Well, if a child became sick the school would let me know and I'd either come up and bring them home or arrange for a taxi to bring them home. When it was raining, I'd try to get other mothers to come and give my kids a ride to school.'

On a very practical level, Heidi advises, 'If you are going out with children, use wrist to wrist bands, or a leash which you hold or attach to your belt. Alternatively, as children grow older, get them to hold hands with a rule that they don't move unless they are all holding hands.'

On Partners

People in general inevitably have issues in a relationship over time; when blindness is factored in, adjustments to a new life are added to the mix. Your partner has to come to terms with your vision loss, which means they have to accept vision loss. There may also be hidden issues of grief, blame, guilt or stigma — for example, at the height of the romantic stage, a partner might initially say that he or she accepts your low vision, but later not be happy seeing you with a white cane or low vision badge. This topic needs to be discussed early on.

Remember, you can't control all matters, you need to ask for help and this requires you to feel comfortable within yourself. We call this acceptance!

Partners and Domestic Violence

I discussed the vulnerability of people with vision impairment to assault in Chapter 17, on Orientation and Mobility. Here, I'll talk specifically about domestic violence.

Very few facts are available on the extent of domestic violence within relationships of people with sight loss, although Australian Government and other agency records suggest this problem is increasing. However, in discussing 'partners,' some principles are worth noting.

- The power imbalance is a major cause of most cases of domestic violence.
1. Domestic violence is not just physical; it can include, emotional and financial imbalance, and issues of daily coercive control. For example, a partner monitoring expenses, phone contacts and friendships. Injury to pets, locking children out of the house, sleep deprivation, sexual abuse, degrading insults, verbal abuse, put-downs based on intelligence or parental capacity, isolation, economic abuse, spiritual abuse, deprivations and denigration of culture, or mis-treatment of pets.
2. Do not ignore early signs. Take action, even though this is often complicated by access to alternative accommodation, finance and a desire to try and make a relationship work. A common belief is that he or she will change.
3. Women and children can display resilience in recovering from domestic violence if specialised services are available.

4. Domestic violence has long-term serious negative psychological, emotional, social and developmental impacts on children.[160]
5. More than one million children in Australia are affected.[161]

On Having Children if You Are Vision Impaired

Like all new parents, parents with vision impairment have no shortage of initial concerns, ranging from feeding and cleaning children to coping with a child's sickness or accidents.

For our friend Heidi whom we have referred to before, the best approach is 'to let go! That is of your reservations, as there is a practical solution to everything'.

If you have partial vision loss, many clients said, practise non-visual skills while you can still see things. Try practising with your eyes shut to understand what it is like to have total sight loss. This also helps build confidence and for you to think about future needs for orientation and mobility support.

Successful parents with vision loss say you have to build up confidence. For example, with nursing and administering medicines, instead of using a teaspoon as most do, transfer medicine from a bottle with a syringe and use a syringe with notches in the handle. You can get such a large syringe from a veterinarian. Don't try to pour liquid from a bottle into a spoon. Alternatively, decant some liquid first into a larger container, then spoon it out, for example a teaspoon is generally regarded as 5 milliliters, three teaspoons make a Table Spoon.

When sighted children are leaving toys around and creating a hazard, tell them that if they leave them on the carpet 'it's gone and

I mean it!' Or, use a broom to sweep toys up to a central point rather than feel for them. Maribel Steel, who lost her sight with retinitis pigmentosa, over a period of years still managed separation from her partner and raised four sighted children. Maribel said on parenting, 'Of course, I suffered from normal parental anxiety but I grew in confidence by learning to listen, to intuit, to smell and to touch when deciding on the best ways to care for my children.

'Naturally, my friends voiced their concerns: "Aren't you afraid your daughter will fall off the play equipment? What if your son runs out onto the road or needs you to remove a splinter? How can you clean a wound from their grazed knee? How do you manage?" I did it with the collective help of my husband, close relatives, friends and the wider community who all pitched in.'[162]

As noted earlier, the reactions of sighted friends are usually based upon disbelief, an apprehension that they could not understand how they themselves could manage. They cast these fears into their responses towards you.

On parenting, Maribel says, 'It was an unexpected gift to view life through my child's eyes, as a whole new world opened up, expanding my confidence as a capable vision-impaired mother, learning to adapt to life with a sighted family. With Claire's eagerness to run up and down the house on countless missions, her life was never dull. I encouraged my daughter to come to me at regular intervals, and tried to turn my dependence on her visual assistance into a game of hide and seek.'[163]

On Genetics

Many causes of early childhood vision loss can be attributed to genetics, which bring about serious blame, guilt, self-doubt, grief and disappointment to parents, as well as requiring explanation, understanding and knowledge.

Genetic testing can provide information about how health or illness is passed on within your family. This knowledge, while vitally important, may also affect your emotional wellbeing, causing stress, anxiety or depression. Some genetic testing can also determine how people are related, which can sometimes show that a person was adopted or that their biological parent is someone other than their legal parent. If these facts were not known previously, they could be troubling. Genetic counselling should therefore be sought to help you understand the nature and implications of your own and your family's genetic findings.[164]

An enlightened approach will require all a family, even the extended family, to undertake genetic testing. Today this is readily available and free through Australia's Medicare and public hospital systems. To find out about this, contact the genetic advice service of your state's public hospital system. You should not have to pay for this test.

A major reason for undertaking genetic testing is that new techniques of gene therapy are now curing young children and preventing progression of genetic diseases in adults. If you know the locus of your affected gene/s, if gene therapy emerges, you will be well placed to either volunteer for trials, or be an early participant in treatment. Genetic testing is now free through

Medicare and your public hospital. To repeat, you will need to undertake genetic counselling.

However, the question of what to tell your child does raise some ethical issues. Depending upon age of the child, the nature of impact, ethnic, cultural or religious values. Genuine questions of what do we say and when, can be problematic. Being too honest or overly dramatising the effect could create a negative outlook for the child. The dilemma of having children if a genetic cause is known, or pre-natal testing, can present difficult challenges, ethical issues for some and very expensive options.[165]

Author Sheila Hocken's family were affected by congenital cataracts causing very blurred vision. In her memoir Emma and I, she writes, 'No one ever talked about blindness, or not being able to see properly, it was accepted as a fact of life and no one mentioned it. Perhaps my mother and father kept up a sort of conspiracy of silence about it for the benefit of Graham and me and if that was so, it was wise. What purpose could it have served to tell a boy and a girl that they were not like other children. We were spared not having our confidence clouded in this way. Falling down and colliding with things had always been so much a part of my life, that I accepted it.'[166]

But in other instances, as mentioned earlier in Chapter 5, guilt and blame can divide a family, leading to the child feeling guilty about their parents' disputes. Such guilt can cause lasting grief and insecurity.

Understanding the impact of a genetic disease does allow a family full consideration of likely future impact and making appropriate changes. For example, being able to intervene in a child's development and education at an early stage with a common-sense approach for lifestyle, work and study choices required for a child's future directions can only be positive. An underlying assumption behind not telling a child about a genetic disease is that there is something bad or shameful about disability — the 'stigma' effect.

As all should, but often don't, to hold an enlightened view that there is nothing wrong with diversity and disability is the best starting point. All humans have, in some way, imperfect genes, and a person's character, personality and potential to contribute to society should not be overlooked — being judged upon the 'content of your character'! Preparing a child for possible stigma or bullying must be part of this enlightenment.

Despite reservations we might feel in taking this informed approach, ultimately it is knowledge that holds the key to empowerment.

On genetics, the ever-pragmatic Heidi says, 'With a genetic condition that's likely to affect your children, it obviously must be discussed with your partner of course. Don't be afraid, it can be a positive fact! If your children have a genetic condition, I think it is important that you prepare them. Say to yourself that children's vision loss is also their training wheels for (hopefully not) blindness. If you see your vision loss experience as training, then you will see it all in a more positive light.'

Communicating with Children, Partners and Friends

If you have vision loss, communication with partners, carers, family and friends depends very much upon your acceptance of your condition and confidence in managing tasks at home. For this reason, when I counsel parents with visual impairment, as an important first step I focus upon the parents' acceptance of vision loss. A person with blindness may still dwell upon their misfortune, remain angry and be too ready to blame others. Not a good start!

As reported in 2009 in the Journal of Visual Impairment and Blindness, 'Since much of the communication between parents and young children is conducted visually, parents who are vision impaired must use other modes of communication. Young children were found to adapt readily to alternate forms of communication for interacting with and developing relationships with their parents who were vision impaired.'[167]

While the role of adaptive technology will contribute to a family's success, simple and cheap solutions also exist. For example, the practice of attaching a bell to a child's clothing so that you know where they are, is successfully adopted by many parents with vision loss. Jacqueline from Victoria, a nearly blind mother, said, 'I carried my children around in a papoose and placed a bell on them and on their socks so I could hear where they were. You learn to worry when there is silence!' Other parents use a restraint harness to keep a child prone to running away within their control.

An often deeply felt question is, 'What is the point of me, as a vision impaired parent, going to watch my child play sport?' The entirely sensible view endorsed by Professor Ron McCallum in his book Born at the Right Time, is that 'It is your support and presence which is so important. Get friends or other parents to tell you about your child's performance and you can comment upon this when he or she comes up afterwards. Until you explain your needs to fellow parents, they will not necessarily know how to convey information back to you.'[168]

I endorse Ron's views. From my experience, while the sports field or swimming pool might only be a total blur and children mere blobs (or perhaps only sounds), if informed by others watching as to what is happening, you can participate and pass comments such as, 'Ken and Fred told me what a great kick you did in the third quarter!' or 'That was a great swim!' or 'Did it hurt much when you fell ...!' Such comments allow you to connect with and share your child's experience even if you haven't seen it. This is not deceptive; you don't have to say, 'I 'saw it!' There's nothing wrong with telling your child that 'Fred told me!' Your child will not be judgemental. It is your acknowledgment, care, love and, above all, your participation children seek and you the beneficiary of their enjoyment/zeal.

Training Children with Vision Loss

With a child who has vision loss, encouraging his or her independence, use of aids and equipment and establishing supportive friendships are typical primary issues which run alongside educational objectives. (See Chapter 15, Schooling Issues.)

As mentioned in Chapter 1, people who are blind at birth will have perception and cognitive issues as the brain's visual cortex does not develop. However, for the majority of children with partial sight loss, Educational Psychologist Geoff Bowen says, 'Fundamentally, "children with vision impairment" have the same range of abilities, personalities and basic needs as their fully sighted classmates. There is no reason why nearly all children with vision impairment should not be placed in the regular classroom and follow the same academic program as other children. Most of them can see, although not well, so that while methods of instruction need to be adapted, there is no need for overall content or aims to differ from the regular program. In fact, it has been stated many times by blind people that the biggest obstacle to their living and learning naturally is the attitude of other people who have normal vision.'[169]

From another perspective, US vision impaired educator and writer Barbara Pierce, states, 'When a blind child enters a family, be it by birth, accident, vision disorder, or adoption, parents and the others close to the youngster face the challenge of supplying the information and concepts that sighted children naturally acquire by visual observation.'[170]

As a general principle, parents should not expect school or other 'experts' to take over the task of developing independence skills. Parents are the ones who can most effectively teach the skills and train habits which enable their child to fit into the family and make friends in the school.

Barbara Pierce also makes the point that parents should not assume that 'children with vision impairment don't need to understand gestures ... facial expressions find their way into the voice.' Parents can assist their child to understand facial gestures such as smiling and frowning by allowing them to feel what they are. They should also know about gestures such as waving.[171]

As earlier mentioned, it is all too easy for parents to over-protect their child with vision impairment, or take the view, 'Oh, it's much quicker if I do it!' Based upon reports from the experience of people who are totally blind, it is best to train children with vision impairment to do up zippers, tie their shoes, fasten buttons, make a bed, polish shoes, pour a glass of milk or unlock a door. As with adults referred to in Chapter 5, there is no need to create learned helplessness. This is one of the key messages I wish to convey in this book: that you do not have to see to do things! This applies to adults as well as children.

If you are a sighted parent of a vision impaired child, don't take over even if you feel rushed and need to get moving. For practice, try to do a task without looking and recognise what parts of the task are most recognisable by touch. This will help you pass on this information to your child. Children do not and should not live in a social vacuum and sighted siblings should not be recruited to protect or shield them. As mentioned earlier, with the Gleeson, Jolley andHingson families, children with vision impairment should be encouraged to join in the fun, to undertake chores as well as play games which build up strength and confidence.

Typical issues encountered include:

- A child's acceptance of disability, and his or her capacity to respond to schoolyard comments such as 'Why do you use a cane?' or 'Why do you look funny?'
- The need to explain disability to others, parents, teachers etc.
- Dealing with inquisitive do-gooders and trying to explain what you or your child can, or cannot see.
- Dealing with other parents.
- Dealing with your feelings of guilt, shame, denial or over-protectiveness.

The following tips that may assist parents considering how they might prepare a child to play are from Barbara Pierce:.

'If your child is blind, or seriously vision impaired, make a game of determining by sound what toy another child is playing with. Balls, blocks, cars, and noise-making pull toys all make distinctive sounds. When a child becomes familiar with his own talking or musical toys, these too are easy to identify.

'One helpful trick is to tie a small bell to the shoe of a playmate who is too young to identify himself reliably when asked. In this way your blind child will know where other children are in the room.

'This information is important for maintaining an accurate idea of what is going on. It is not easy to strike a balance between urging the blind child to enter into play with others and providing her with the quiet stream of information that helps orient her to her surroundings. Each child will make progress at his or her own rate. What is enough information for one child to get started and continue independently is not sufficient for another.'[172]

Some more ideas to encourage participation are worth considering:

- Use a larger ball.
- Encourage hopping rather than skipping.
- Invite a group of playmates to your place to play.
- Offer refreshments whenever playmates gather at your place.

Also, if play equipment is fun, not only will other children want to play, but the blind child will be encouraged to learn to move and take part.

It may be even more important for blind children than for sighted to learn early the first rules of successful social engagement, for example:

- Don't bite.
- Share your toys.
- Engage in appropriate conversation.
- Do not echo or use imitative speech patterns.
- Give other people a chance to talk.
- Don't rock (rocking is a typical characteristic seen where spacial orientation cannot be intuitive).
- Look at the speaker.

Working on these and similar points of acceptable conduct will improve the chances that a vision impaired child will make friends. I guess that the following ideal applies to all child raising, but, getting a child to learn how to behave considerately and politely takes tenacity on the part of parents and hard work on the part of blind children, but the benefits last a lifetime. Remember, don't wait until it's too late, praise yourself when even getting little things right!

Issues of Grief for Parents

The grief responses referred to in earlier chapters apply with parents of children with vision impairment. Parents may have prior expectations for their child and now hold a tension between what might have been an what is now emerging. Parents may have to deal with loss, the concept that a disabled child is 'a death of a child which should have been'. In interviewing a father from an Italian background about his totally blind boy's potential for study, Margaret Fialides from the RVIB said, 'Mr.

'X' just broke down in tears. I think it was the first time that he had shared the grief over loss of his son's sight!'[173]

The loss of dreams, fantasies, comparisons to other children and the normal celebrations of a child's life and development through school can contribute to unresolved grief and Post Traumatic Stress Syndrome (PTSS),[174] which has been identified to exist among 20 per cent of vision impaired mothers.[175]

The typical responses of denial, referred to earlier, as applying to those with vision loss, also apply to parents as part of normal coping. Encouraging independence, awareness of the impact on siblings and of ethnic and cultural differences are important considerations, which are best dealt with where there is openness, no denial. To keep parents happy and well-adjusted is important for family health, but adjustment to disability as noted earlier, can be ongoing.

(15)

Schooling Issues

'Tell me and I forget, teach me and I may remember, involve me and I learn.'

Benjamin Franklin

'I have never let my schooling interfere with my education.'

Mark Twain

Why this Chapter?

This chapter has been prepared once again as a result of the numerous issues raised in discussion groups I conducted for parents. The issues they raised were always complex and compelling, and parents always showed a great thirst for knowledge. As will be immediately recognized, this area is highly specialized and I do not attempt to provide more than a summary of key issues. I have also tried here to address some schooling issues by quoting and paraphrasing the ideas and advice of experts in the field of disability education.

Identifying Vision Loss in Children

It was not until I was in Grade Five of primary school that my pre-RP eye condition of Myopia was noticed by my teacher. Up until then, I had become very adept at peering over my desk mate's shoulder to see answers. As a consequence, I never truly understood mathematics. At one stage prior to being exposed for this fraud, I had been given the illustrious task of bell ringer for the school. I had no wristwatch, so the Headmaster, at that stage oblivious to my Myopia, hung a stop watch up on the wall of the external locker room. When asked if I could read it, I just said 'yes!' However, to read this watch I had to literally jump up to see the watch's face, or rely upon friends to tell me. As soon as my so-called friends read the time, they, to my intense annoyance, rushed off and rang the bell themselves. This lasted until one day, forgetting time altogether, I rang the bell 20 minutes late only to be summarily dismissed.

Notwithstanding my experience, teachers may be the first to identify that a child has difficulties with vision. The number with vision difficulties can be as high as 'one in five' of all children in early years where Myopia is undetected. Unsurprisingly, refractive errors causing difficulty in reading and attaining satisfactory literacy levels have a major impact on academic achievement. Such vision problems can usually be addressed with corrective glasses and/or minor modifications in the classroom.

There are certain behaviours or characteristics that may also alert a teacher to the fact that a student may have vision problems. These include:

- the appearance of the eyes — turned, red, teary, or excessive blinking
- complaints — headaches, dizziness, blurry, watery eyes or light sensitivity
- behavioural aspects — head turning across the page, head tilted to one side, holding books very close to the face, looking at a fellow student's work, frequently rubbing eyes, becoming irritated when completing written work
- eye movement — losing place when reading, using a finger to track the words, omitting small words, writing up or down on the paper
- eye coordination — seeing double, repeating letters, misaligning digits, squinting, tilting their head, poor eye–hand coordination, or feeling objects
- refractive — difficulty copying from board to paper.

While one might think that technology and adaptive software is revolutionising access for people with vision loss, research confirms most children already spend more than three hours watching TV and perhaps as high as six hours a day before screens.[176] The use of smaller, portable screens mean closer viewing distances, which increases demand on the eye to accommodate the image. It is understood this may have detrimental effects for some eye conditions. There have also been concerns that as access to digital technology and screen time increases, so does the potential for increased vision problems. Visual fatigue occurs when eye muscles tighten during visually intense tasks, which causes the muscles to become uncomfortable and eyes dry and irritated.

As a matter of general information, in considering the types of vision loss encountered at schools, education Psychologist Geoff Bowen, of the Victorian Statewide Vision Resource Centre (SVRC),[177] notes that:

- it is estimated that 70–80 per cent of everything we learn depends upon sight with consequential impact upon social, emotional, behavioural and learning abilities.
- multiple problems are more common in children with congenital visual impairment than in children who become visually impaired later on.
- 60–80 per cent of children have multiple disabilities.
- about 75 per cent of visual impairments result from some problem with aspects of the central nervous system, such as retinopathy of primaturity, and about 25 per cent of visual impairments result from a 'mechanical' problem of the eye, such as glaucoma, congenital cataracts, colobomas, aniridia, progressive myopia.[178]

Some Negative School Experiences

As we know, discrimination at school is not limited to blindness. In primary school my boy, who has dyslexia, was shamed before his class when asked by his teacher, who knew of this disability, to stand up in front of the class and read aloud from a book.

Of course, he could not do so and he, like many others who experience disadvantage at school, found the negative experience intensely traumatic and long-lasting.

One of the most distressing stories coming out of my discussion groups involved a mother with near total vision loss. Wendy from Queensland, with diabetic retinopathy, in tears, told the group, 'I found that other parents shunned me and my boy. When I asked school friends of my son to come over to my home for his birthday, I know some mothers would not let their children come as they thought that as I was a blind person it wouldn't be safe! Then I found they didn't ask my boy to their parties in return. It was so hurtful I just cried and cried for days!'

Successful vision impaired parents report that problems such as engagement by Wendy in the greater school community can be overcome. The pathway to success here involves that old chestnut: educating those around you to develop an understanding that blindness is not to be feared, nor are people with sight loss helpless and hopeless. This requires sufficient self-esteem and confidence, but if you as an individual are still struggling with adjustment and acceptance, such a task will appear overwhelming. Some initial steps to deal with this challenge as advised by successful parents, could include:

- Find out if there are other parents with vision loss in the school community.
- Talk to the principal and class teachers, understand the school's curriculum and the school's attitudes to inclusiveness. Many school Mission Statements refer to their 'Pastoral Care'. How this is provided needs to be explored.

Assess the principal's sincerity in addressing disability issues and if you feel ill at ease, select another school if possible.

- Ask a service provider such as Guide Dogs or Vision Australia if there are educational or child psychology specialists available, are there relevant children and parents support groups or mentors you can speak with.
- Gain the support of an Orientation and Mobility Specialist, or school welfare support to give tips to you and your school community to assist with settling in.

On dealing with this difficult issue of fitting in, Joanne, a mother from New South Wales with keratoconus,[179] said, 'I found the best thing was to get involved in the school committees and the Tuck Shop. It allowed both teachers and parents to understand that, although I used a cane, I wasn't totally useless!' This view was supported by most who had gone through the school 'experience'.

A vision impaired parent with nystagmus — involuntary, rapid movement of the eyes — reported on the lack of support she received from the headmaster and teachers. 'I know they were all looking at me with my funny eyes and treating me as if I were stupid!' said Mary from Queensland who later took legal action against the school for discrimination. Taking positive action, she took her children out of that school. (My group's suggestion at the time was for her to wear sunglasses when talking with staff to cover up her eye defect, provided it was safe to do so.)

Questions to Ask about Your Child

1. What are my child's strengths and weaknesses? What are some examples of each strength or weakness?

2. Does my child participate, speak or ask questions during the class and in any of the classroom activities?

3. For the most part, does my child seem happy and to be adjusting well to school?

4. Is my child getting along with others? Are there any classroom relationships or situations which I need to be made aware of?

5. Have you noticed any changes in behaviour that I should be concerned with? Is my child complaining of having trouble seeing the board or does my child seem sleepy?

6. Does my child work up to his or her potential?

7. How does my child approach test taking?

8. What are some of the upcoming subjects the students will be studying, and how might we support these units from home?

9. Does my child understand the expectations of this classroom?

10. Is my child turning homework in on time?

11. Is there an action plan we can develop to keep improving my child's progression?[180]

Some General Approaches

It appears that the better view of psychologists and educators[181] is that presentations of 'blindness awareness' within the classroom is to be encouraged for children with sight so that they understand the tools and techniques to be used for vision loss and not fear blindness.

To start with, children with vision loss lack visual and

response cues normally found with socialisation, of which some aspects include:

- understanding peer group norms and participation
- understanding body language
- understanding risk taking
- cooperation and sharing.

All of the above can be affected with vision loss. Encouraging students with normal sight to understand, support and work with students with vision impairment is part of a teacher's role.

From a parent's point of view, Barbara Pierce, writer and educator from the National Federation of the Blind in the USA (NFB), says, 'Encourage your child to become active in a school or extracurricular program. If you don't hear your child mention the names of classmates or kids from, for example, church, sport, or Scouts, probe to learn why not. Be creative in constructing opportunities for friendships to grow.'[182] If they are not happening, look for the explanation, and by liaising with your child's teacher work out a strategy of what your child can do about it. Maybe this requires education of the class by a specialist or other person with vision impairment.

Parents with vision loss often achieve the above goal by successfully arranging to visit a class with their Dog Guide, cane and simulation glasses so that classmates for their child can experience and understand what vision loss means. At a recent school visit, Susie Barrington from Sydney was asked by children, 'How do you know your Dog Guide likes you?' Susie, who was seated, called her dog Tilley over and said 'Show Mumma you love her!' Tilly then placed her paws around Susie's neck as if to cuddle), reached up and licked Susie's face, to the shrieks of delight, laughter and universal applause of the class. Most schools are happy to support such initiatives, well, perhaps not dogs licking faces!

A parent or teacher can also arrange to use cardboard simulation glasses, which mimic types of vision loss, thereby assist people with sight to comprehend what partial sight really means. A parent, teacher of vision impaired children, or blind adult can make blindness seem less scary, even interesting. However, Barbara Pierce says, 'adults can't make classmates do more than give the blind student a chance to make a place for himself or herself'.

Based upon the experience of Orientation and Mobility Specialists and of blind mentors such as Susie Barrington, it remains important to consider when demonstrating white canes, simulation glasses and other aids or equipment, to ensure this experience for sighted children is not creating fear or negativity about sight loss. Demonstrations of this kind should highlight the skills and trust required in using aids and importance for mobility, but this is not helpful if sighted pupils are left feeling blindness is scary, or sad. Such demonstrations should engender acceptance and understanding for others.

Some Principles for Educating Children with Vision Impairment

NOTE: The topic of education, and particularly of educating children with vision loss, is too specialised and complex to be given justice here. However, as general guidance, I attempt to summarise key concepts often referred to by educationalists and psychologists. Some principles include:

- It is understood that children in general develop and learn cumulatively, starting from birth.
- Early learnt skills form the basis for further development.
- Behaviour and functioning are influenced by the immediate social and physical environment.
- If warm and responsive caregiving is provided, positive attachments will develop, providing a secure basis for learning.
- Children with disabilities initiate interactions less frequently.
- Children with disabilities give subtle cues which are difficult to read.
- Caregivers and providers must become skilled observers of the cues given to create secure attachments and effective relationships.
- Providing mainstream education now accepted as 'essential', requires provision of additional secure supports to gain the same benefits as for sighted children.[183]

The concept of inclusiveness is a key objective of the teaching experience with children who have a disability. Australian educators Melissa Cain and Melissa Fanshawe state that 'Being inclusive of students with disabilities in the classroom, helps all students develop empathy and understanding for their peers. It is important to note that designing learning activities for all students does not mean designing for the average student. In fact, studies demonstrate that when you design for the average, the outcomes usually suits no one. Classrooms can be designed to suit the individual needs of all students which will encourage active participation for students with vision impairment.'[184]

Cain and Fanshawe go on to recommend that teachers provide students with 'a toolbox of technologies, both digital and traditional, to help access the curriculum. An Expanded Core curriculum helps compensate for vision loss. For children with mild or moderate vision impairment, modify content in the least restrictive manner and create an inclusive culture promoting active participation of all students.'

Academic Impacts of Vision Impairment

It is widely reported that vision impairment creates a particular challenge in the Australian mainstream classroom, as the content and the assessment of the curriculum is designed for those who can see. Visual images are used throughout classrooms and schools in the form of posters, signs and displays. Multimedia is embedded throughout the national curriculum with many visual images and videos, models and symbols for students to decode. Subjects such as Science, Mathematics, Geography, History and Visual Art have proved infinitely more difficult to access by students with low vision. These subjects contain a high number of graphical representations, diagrams, graphs, tables and pictorial representation of data.

Research in several Western countries has revealed that students with vision impairment often feel lonely and isolated from their peers. Students do not like to perceive themselves as different, particularly in the teenage years, and using white canes or reading Braille highlights such differences. In her book Emma and I, Sheila Hocken writes, 'I had no idea that I couldn't see normally until I was about seven. I lived among vague images and colours which were blurred, as if a gauze were over them and I thought that was how everybody else saw the world ... even in my dreams the people had no faces.'[185]

In attempting to fit in with others while experiencing partial vision loss which is not immediately obvious, a child may develop intense avoidance characteristics. There may be difficulties in participating in sports. Janet Shaw in Beyond the Red Door, makes the point that teachers are often afraid that a child with vision impairment will be hurt and unable to compete, which then leads to excluding vision impaired children from games, which leads to further feelings of exclusion and difference on the part of the children'.[186]

Classroom Communications for Children with Vision Impairment

As noted earlier, a sighted observer naturally finds it hard to adjust their own senses to notice textures, sounds, shapes and odours (See Chapters 4, 5 and 17) Call attention to nonvisual cues which are also relevant for general orientation. (See Chapter 17 on Orientation and Mobility.)

US early childhood development and education philosophy[187] considers that, as can be expected, the normal facial or hand gestures of a teacher may have little effect for a child with vision loss. Pity, as discussed earlier in this book, should be avoided and a teacher is required to provide a greater level of clear verbal instructions. Lowering your voice rather than raising it when giving instructions and, above all, praising students for their cooperation and success, is essential. Clear boundaries need to be set and enforced.

Things to Look for with Schools

If you're a parent of a vision impaired child, make sure you ask yourself these questions when your child starts school:

- 'Selecting the school — how will my child fit in/manage? In country or regional areas, will a child's vision loss be supported?
- How do I introduce the subject of my children with disability to the school and friends? This means understanding your child's needs and what they can and cannot see.
- What do I say to teachers and what to do if a teacher displays intolerance, or perceived lack of respect? Not all schools or teachers are supportive. In one example, when a vision impaired mother found a teacher could not or would not control teasing of her children, and the principal was also unhelpful, she took her children out to change schools. An approach of some under-resourced government schools may be to let the 'problem' children go to another neighbourhood school as an easy option. The following may provide some guidance,
- How do I identify school problems with my child and read my child's responses correctly? Also, what disability supports are there in the education system? What technology exists; how do I fund it? What training support is there? Dealing with the educational institutions — barriers such as, rules, study

systems and study techniques, coaching and mentoring, will form part of the journey.

- Am I willing to ask for help in the school environment and deal with discrimination within the school — whether it be from children, teachers, parents or principals — yes, it does happen! However, becoming accepted within the school environment is important. Joining the Tuck Shop and school committees can work to accomplish this.

PART THREE:

Some Practical Solutions

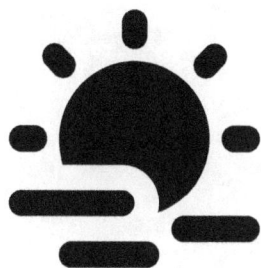

Some Practical Solutions

(16)

Independence in the Home, Community and Kitchen

'I am no bird; and no net ensnares me: I am a free human being with an independent will.'

Charlotte Brontë, Jane Eyre

'The most courageous act is still to think for yourself — Aloud!'

Coco Chanel

Remaining at Home

In many discussion groups where the question of remaining at home was discussed, a frequently expressed concern was, 'My children want me to go into an aged care home. They think I can't look after myself!' On further questioning and discovering that the client was not frail, isolated and otherwise experiencing mobility or cognitive issues, I advised, 'Well, blindness is not the reason to leave your home.' In providing this advice, I was also guided by the comments of many who had gone into aged care at their children's insistence, that they 'hated it' and 'wished they had remained in their former home and neighbourhood'. Isolation and loneliness were key factors.

It is my firm view that maintaining our independence in the home is the first step in creating confidence. It allows you to keep your privacy, remain comfortable with pre-existing skills and familiarity with your environment, and keep your attachment with positive memories and friendships while remaining in control. From this starting point, people with vision impairment will be more able to venture into the community with confidence.

Of course, much depends upon whether or not you are single, or have other illnesses. Often a caring partner is there to provide support. However, while I'm not saying this is at all wrong, it still remains important that, rather than relying on a partner to do everything ('smother love'), you retain confidence and capacity to cook and maintain your home in the unhappy event that your partner might predecease you, or become incapable of looking after you.

I recommend that you can consider these five critical factors:

1. Do you have sufficient skills, capacity and interest to keep on shopping, maintaining finances, cooking and maintaining self-care?
2. Do you access community activities, church or social groups? Perhaps you are quite happy living alone.

3. Do you have good neighbours or pre-existing home care supports?
4. Are you physically isolated from shops and amenities, or have poor mobility with limited access to public transport?
5. Are you interested in and willing to take up using gadgets and technology?

In addition to a federal government policy, which encourages keeping older generations in their own home as a more cost-effective public policy option, a majority of Australians prefer to remain in their own home.[188] A better psychological outcome tends to result when living in an environment with memories, friends, garden and a familiar neighbourhood.

Preparing to Stay Home

If you are determined to remain at home, ask yourself these questions:

- How recent is your sight loss, what is the cause and how is it affecting you?
- Do you have a family nearby and willing to support you, or do you know of service agencies for vision impairment who can assist you to make your home safe?
- What tasks can you do without difficulty?
- What are tasks where you might need some small assistance?
- What are tasks you have great difficulty with?
- How will you explain your difficulties, to whom and what words will you use? Perhaps it will be helpful to get your family or

friends to use simulation glasses to let them understand what you can and cannot see.

- How can you make it clear to everyone that it is very important for you to continue with your existing lifestyle? Other blind people remain independent and unless there are other mobility, isolation or disability issues, there is no reason why you can't!

- What organisational systems or gadgets could you use? Many are listed in Chapter 18 (Technology and Working in the Shed). Talk to other vision impaired people or support staff in service organisations to find out what is available. It is as simple as a phone call!

If you have difficulty in using the phone and looking up phone numbers, either change to smartphones, a large print phone with some memory functions. Otherwise, get training and support, which will empower you to use your phone. Remember, if people who are totally blind and aged in their 90s can do this, so can you.

Organisation, a Key Principle

When it comes to organising ourselves and our surroundings, what suits one person may not suit another; our vision loss can be as different as our needs. The following tips are based on what clients have identified:

- Be organised, slow down and be prepared to spend more time planning your tasks and daily activities.
- De-clutter and simplify your surrounds and garden, or get help.

- De-clutter your mind! This includes removing grief and attachment to objects you no longer use or need.

The great principle I have found for myself and gained confidence from, is initially hard to accept, but it is that you do not have to use sight to remain independent! In addition to smart technology, the use of touch, smell, hearing and taste allow us to function successfully. Experience creates the required trust. Your hands and touch 'become your eyes!'

Apart from using smart technology, to overcome frustrations of trying to see, keep things identified with tactile (touch) markers. You can use simple, low-cost items such as rubber bands (by placing one band around an identical item); and for wet areas, Velcro, plastic bubbles, Puff Paint, or other adhesive water-proof strips such as Croc Grip tape.

Tactile markers can be used on stoves, microwaves, washing machines and other objects, even keyboards or phone buttons.

Alternatively, in labelling items, use technology such as a Pen Friend organiser, or apps on smartphones such as Seeing AI for iPhones, or Supersense AI for Androids, to read print. If you have some useable sight, then using a CCTV, or other scanning or reading device, needs consideration, although access in the kitchen may present difficulties.

For the common problem of identifying similar looking objects such as hair shampoo and conditioner bottles, place a rubber band around one of the pair.

Another solution to a problem most people find vexing is, placing toothpaste on your brush. Well, don't! Place toothpaste on your finger or directly in your mouth! Get your own tube of toothpaste if required.

There is a large range of clocks, watches and timers which help — see the equipment listed below. This includes lighting. Getting an occupational therapist to assist you here is important.

If you cannot afford a new gadget, ask your family to assist by buying you presents for Mother's/Father's Day, birthdays or Christmas. That way, you can assemble useful devices such as a Pen Friend organiser, CCTV scanners, talking scales, and so on. (See Chapter 18.) This is also a good way to satisfy family members who want to help, but do not know how to, or do not know what might be useful. Your family will feel good they are helping out.

Many people now rely on smart technology tablets, but desktop or laptop computers still remain great organisers. Set yourself up at home with a tablet or computer which has text-to-speech functionality.

For handling mail and paying bills, if you are a smartphone user, use apps such as Seeing AI or Supersense AI, or if you use a computer, get a printer/scanner and extra software connected to it to read your typed (not handwritten) mail so you can respond by email, and also keep information such as copies of documents, letters and recipes.

Finally, apps such as AIRA and 'be my eyes' offer a person who can read, or identify items for you. AIRA has fees.

Safety in the Home

There are more accidents in the home than anywhere else, even for people who are sighted! Therefore, it is vital for everyone with vision impairment to develop and maintain increased safety habits in and around the home. This is especially true for those at the commencement of vision loss where you are used to rushing around, perhaps doing several tasks at once. First principle: slow down and plan/organise what you want to do.

The suggestions below are based upon general rules for safety; follow them to eliminate hazards and be safe:

- Eliminate small throw rugs; they can cause tripping.
- Make sure your bath mat has a non-skid backing.
- Keep electrical cords as close to the baseboards as possible and out of walkways.
- Keep floor lamps and small items such as low tables, magazine racks and plants out of walkways.
- Label cleaning and toxic products with tactile markers to make them easily identifiable, and store them and any flammable or combustible items away from the kitchen or heating units.
- Plugging a cord into an electrical outlet is a great cause of frustration. Here's how to line the plug up with the sockets. Use some Velcro to make two small arrows and while the cord is plugged in, match them up, one on top of the socket and the other on top of the plug. You will be amazed how simple this task then becomes when matching these arrows.
- Clean up spills immediately. If you forget the spill is there, you might slip on it. Don't panic! Divide the soiled area up into smaller simulated squares, and clean them one by one. Gail, former Executive Officer of Blind Citizens Australia (BCA), who had severe vision loss, once had a cleaning job in a rather posh suburb for a haughty lady, who asked her to clean a large mirror in her lounge room. 'I panicked at

first,' said Gail, 'but then adopted a method of dividing the mirror into a series of hypothetical squares. When I had finished, in trepidation I called in the lady. "Oh, what a great job!" cried the matriarch. "The lady who did it last time must have been blind!"

In cleaning up an area, a sensible approach is, don't make large rapid sweeps, divide the area up into smaller areas, sweep slowly to a bench or wall, or corner. Maureen, from New South Wales, a discussion group participant said, 'I dropped some glass and as I was in bare feet and afraid of cutting myself, all I could do was sit up on top of my kitchen bench for three hours until my partner came home!'

Keep practising skills and remember to close cabinet, wardrobe and cupboard doors and drawers as soon as you've taken out what you need. Open doors remain a real and serious danger at any height!

Practice until it becomes second nature, to hold one arm out in front of your head when bending down, or body when approaching cupboards. Make this an essential practice.

Install smoke, fire and carbon monoxide alarms and check the batteries regularly to make sure these devices are still working.

Know where to find your electrical circuit breaker or fuse box and water turn-off valve. Learn how to use them safely.

When visitors call, keep outside doors locked until they have identified themselves to your satisfaction. A strong, lockable wire door is sensible.

In the kitchen and laundry, mark oven settings, and microwave, washing machine and thermostats with tactile markers at the settings you most typically use. Be selective as too many markers can create confusion. Use an occupational therapist or person with sight to assist.

Pick up shoes, clothing, books, and other items that you could trip over. Put away any object in boxes, or use bulldog clips to hold them together as a pair — for example, many people keep shoe boxes for this purpose.

When sorting clothes, use a talking colour detector, colour ID, or a phone app, such as Seeing AI or AIRA or Tap See, or be my eyes. The device Pen Friend has washable tags. A good tactile tip to identify clothes is to sew on buttons, cut off part of the tag, or sew on a thread, etc. Use 'sock pegs' or safety pins to keep socks together.

General Tips for Public Safety

In addition to concerns people with vision impairment may hold, the general rules identified by police for safety in the community should be followed.

If you feel threatened:

1. Do your best to draw the attention of people nearby, scream or call out, or carry a loud personal alarm. These personal alarms are relatively low cost and can usually be found online or perhaps through your Neighborhood Watch.
2. Go to a safe place where there are other people.
3. Be overt and call Triple Zero (000) in Australia. Have emergency numbers in your contact lists, or ask your smartphone's personal assistant to dial.
4. Prepare before you go out. Are you aware of dangerous locations or times of day? Keep valuables out of sight, be

confident, hold your head high and walk confidently, if possible walk on the footpath against the flow of traffic, and be as observant as possible. While not seeing detail, you may still be able to identify people in proximity. Try not to be preoccupied with texts, listening to music or talking on your phone. However, using AIRA where a professional assistant can describe your environment, could be helpful. AIRA offers a free 5 minute service which could help in an emergency.

5. If you see, or hear suspicious characters, or situations, stay at a distance and call for help rather than 'toughing it out'.

6. Most opportunist thieves want easy pickings: smartphones, purses, computers, bags etc. Always carry your mobile phone out of sight. Even if you have no provider connection, you can still dial an emergency number. In Australia, this is 112. This is not to be confused with the 000 number used for emergencies.

7. If listening to music, keep one ear free to listen to your environment.

8. Use well-lit roads at night, and avoid unlit paths and streets. If you travel a regular route, vary your route.

In general, staying connected with your community helps you stay confident. Walking out confidently and projecting a positive image of yourself to the world is best.

Orientation in the Home

It may appear surprising, but people with severely reduced sight can get lost even in their home or backyard. Think of it this way, if you had blurry vision, glare and foggy sight, you may lose depth perception, it's quite easy to become disorientated.

In fact, in the house or garden, as totally blind peer Paul Holmes says, 'Use a radio as a good way to orientate yourself by hearing the direction from where it is playing. This works also if you are working in the garden.'

Don't put tools down and then possibly trip on them, place them in safe containers like a wheely bin or wheelbarrow.

Don't panic! Stop and focus on a sound, smell or object.

Many vision impaired people advise that they often become disorientated inside their own home. Sounds silly, doesn't it? But this is surprisingly easy where light or uniform coloured walls exist and no contrast between walls and floor is evident, or in darkness. (See Chapter 17, Orientation and Mobility, for further details.) The following may also assist:

- Train yourself and other family members always to either, shut or leave doors completely open and not to leave them half open. A half-open door presents little contrast and is easy to run into — it is very painful! This applies to cupboard doors; bumping into their sharp edges can hurt. As mentioned, develop a practice to always close a door after opening.
- At night, it is recommended for those with some sight, to use sensor-activated lights within the home and solar lights for pathways and drives.
- Hold your hand outwards so that the outside of your hand brushes the wall. If you use the inner palm or fingers, you might get splinters or cuts, which further limit your ability to touch.

- Have other family members keep walkways clear. Children typically just dump bags, shoes or pullovers and so on, so they must be trained from an early age to respect your needs. You really do have to be assertive here.
- Cleaning and Shopping: get home help, or ask coordinators or volunteers to organise for someone to come and help you with reading, shopping, walking etc. (Note: programs in Australia such as the National Disability Insurance Scheme (NDIS), if you are under 65 years, and My Aged Care (MAC), if you are over 65 years, will cover these supports, but with MAC, expect delays.)

Shopping

If you're experiencing vision loss, you may not feel as safe travelling outside your home to shop as you once did. However, the same safety precautions you've always taken, plus a few extra, still apply. For example, it's best to go slowly. Some people just start by finding their letter box first, then venture out street by street. (See Chapter 17, Orientation and Mobility.)

If you need help, always ask for it; it gets results. Yes it is one of our great challenges, but people will willingly render assistance. There can be credibility issues — for example, 'You don't look blind!' — but using an ID badge or ID cane helps. Remember, sighted people find it hard to understand and accept vision loss.

Your shopping can be delivered, or done online, but if you want to go down the street, don't struggle trying to read items, always ask at the Customer Help Desk for assistance. Supermarkets have free apps that identify the aisle, contents and price of items, and recent advice is that both the Coles and Woolworths apps have improved.

Some people use compact CCTV scanners to read sales tickets, others take a photo with iPhone or Android and enlarge it — the two finger expansive flick! Others use barcode readers as in the App Seeing AI, or dedicated devices, but these methods can be slow. (See Chapter 18, Technology and Working in the Shed.)

It is usually quicker to ask for help from supermarket assistants than to persevere looking for an item. Taking a collapsible shopping trolley, or backpack to carry items home, leaves your arm free for cane or dog. Otherwise arrange for home delivery.

Paying bills is much easier if you use direct debit — but make sure funds are available. You can negotiate monthly direct debits if you take advantage of the fact that you are 'blind'. This also helps with budgeting your cash flow. Saying that you are 'blind' also helps when you want better service. Usually, the company will send you an email or text to remind you of accounts due. Alternatively, use telephone banking. In Australia, cross counter service at a bank usually has no service fees if you are on a pension, but check with your bank and have this noted in their files.

With credit cards in Australia, no pin required for transactions under $A200 with 'Tap and Go'. But if you have to enter your pin, remember telling someone your pin breeches your contract with the bank and makes you vulnerable. A sales point keypad is similar to a landline phone and has a small raised dot on the number 5 key. Other key markings are, a raised circle on the 'OK' button and a raised cross on the 'Cancel' button.

If you are using a pin number at a supermarket or shop, practise first on your standard phone at home. Train yourself not to look;

instead, get the feel of how you can move your fingers around the number 5 key. Like all matters involved with the transition from sight to vision impairment, it takes practice.

The recent introduction of the 'touch pad' funds transfer system is presenting significant difficulties for vision impaired people. Only the introduction of some tactile features or audio will improve this situation. A recent case in Australia's Equal Opportunity Commission found in December 2018, that flat screens with no accessibility features 'are discriminatory'.

When it comes to handling money, you have several options: put the largest denominations to one side of your wallet, get organised at home before you go out, and use only $50 or $20 denominations so you know what the note is when you take it out. Alternatively, fold the $20 bills lengthways and the $50 bills longways. Get a wallet with two separate compartments or use a thick card to separate your notes.

Australian bills all have different lengths and a series of raised dots to distinguish the different denominations. These dots are: — $5, one, $10, two, $20, three, $50, four, and not yet, but eventually $100 — 5.

If you are a smartphone user, get the app, Cash Reader, which costs about A$10 per year or A$28 for lifetime support. This app is excellent and reads banknotes from all countries in the world.

When using coins, you can get the shop assistant to count them, although most people might not trust this method. In an open situation as in a supermarket, you can usually trust the assistant. In most countries, you can identify coin edges which usually have serrated edges with gaps in the serration for higher denominations. Or use coin holders. It is quite practical in your familiar home and local community environment, to ask sales staff, cashiers, or taxi drivers to tell you what the denomination of bank notes are before handing them over. This works on the basis that, if it is too low, you will quickly be told!

In the Kitchen: Cooking Tips

Again, and again, people with vision impairment say, 'I can't cook anymore! Or I now have to order Meals on Wheels!' Of course, there is nothing wrong with getting Meals on Wheels and if you don't want to cook, that's fine. Many women — and yes, it is mostly women — after a lifetime catering for families are only too pleased to be relieved of this role. However, for many, cooking is a great skill, preferred lifestyle, hobby, relaxation or health objective.

So, let's get one principle clear. There is no reason why vision loss prevents you from cooking, but there are a number of important tips to learn.

People who are totally blind can cook and so, if they can, why can't you? As previously mentioned, it is all about doing it differently! Here are some basic tips: -

What to do when you want to follow a recipe? Without a doubt, the Google Home voice-activated devices and others, Mini, Home and Max, are wonderful. Through them, you can request Google to tell you a recipe. Google will then take you through the ingredients and cooking procedure. Elixir and other voice recognition devices provide an excellent, almost unlimited supply of recipes with options on ingredients and cooking instructions. Just ask Google — 'Hey Google, give me a recipe!' — and it will guide you through.

Place the items you intend to use on your kitchen bench in the order of use, placing them against a wall or divider. Try to avoid going back and forward to the pantry and refrigerator to fetch and put back items as this creates a situation that can lead to distraction or mistakes. Have your recipe sorted first using whichever system suits you: Google, a computer, Pen Friend, large print book or tape recorder.

In principle, always pour liquids over the sink, have a cloth ready in case of spillages, know your cooking times and use a timer. A smartphone or Google Home can act as a timer. Just ask Siri (iPhone) or Google to give you a reminder in say, five minutes.

Remember, all cooks burn things, so don't blame your lack of vision for this as organisation is the key. A typical trap is that, while we are waiting for something to boil or cook, we get distracted on the phone or computer. Try to avoid this.

Here are some general cooking and pantry tips:

- Cook on low heat.
- Don't cook too long.
- Use aromas as a guide for identifying herbs and spices and when cooking for when something is over-heating/burning. If you have poor sense of smell, use timers, tactile markers for your heat gauges thermometers and train with an OT.
- When cutting up soft meat like chicken or fish, semi-freeze it first; it becomes more solid and easier to slice.
- When cooking a chop or steak, sear the sides to seal juices; you only need heat when cooking one side. Turn the meat over, turn the heat off and let the residual heat in the pan cook the other side.

- When pouring olive oil, decant some from your tin or larger bottle into a wide glass/plastic jar with a screw-on lid so that you can use a tablespoon to lift pour out the oil as required.
- To guard against cutting yourself, for example when slicing onions or tomatoes, which are hard and slippery, make sure knives are sharp, as blunt knives tend to slip. In holding the tomato or onion, curl any extended fingers back and hold the object with thumb and forefinger knuckle. Place the knife alongside your finger to measure thickness before slicing. You can also obtain devices which slice. Remember, slow down!
- Use contrasting colour cutting boards.
- Use extra lighting and portable under-cupboard lamps, and have glare from windows or overhead light assessed.
- For slicing, use a food processer, and cut into quarters — a manual food processor is sold by the King of Knives shop, which is good for onions, carrots and garlic.
- When it comes to assessing if food is bad, trust your own experience. Use touch or smell. Is it crisp? Or slippery? Or does it feel soft and spongy? Err on the side of caution and dispose of stale food.
- A key skill is organisation. Simplify and de-clutter your work areas. Create space.
- Your pantry requires thought and organisation. You can use rubber bands as a low-cost way to place over objects for ease of identification, especially where two objects are identical. , cut down boxes as a low-cost alternative to more costly storage units, or purchase plastic bins of all shapes and sizes for storage. If you have some sight, use coloured plastic tubs to keep selected items in.

- Use the Pen Friend digital recorder with programmed labels to record your voice and when the Pen Friend is turned on it re-reads what's on the label. To economise, place the label on a magnet or plastic label with rubber band, or plastic lid to place in the freezer for re-use. You can also label medications plus directions, CDs, wine, etc.

- To identify items, use a talking barcode scanner or use apps such as Seeing AI or Supersense AI. AIRA Vision, while expensive, does have a free five-minute service, or the app, be my eyes, where a person will read or identify items for you. (See Chapter 18, Technology and Working in the Shed.)

- In organising your kitchen with useable sight, use colours, but if your sight is not helpful, use tactile aids such as duct tape or Velcro, or plastic stick-on bubbles as tactile markers, or waterproof Croc Grip tape. Band-It tactile bands are brightly coloured stretch bands with differing raised symbols (such as triangles) which you place around objects. You might need a person with sight to initially help you.

- Some kitchen appliances have flat touch screens, in which case use tactile markers if possible. When purchasing appliances, consider all options, explain your vision to the salesman and get them to turn on the machine so you can check the flat screen and other operational features.

- You can buy talking microwaves, induction cook tops, kettles, etc. Check with your blindness Agency shop, or online.

- The shops run by blindness agencies usually have a range of helpful products for the kitchen, including a bread cutting guide, an aid for holding fruit or vegetables in place while they are being cut and an aid for cutting sandwiches.

Cooking Items Recommended by Blind and Vision Impaired Users

The following general cooking items and appliances were recommended by clients in discussion groups. Keep in mind, however, that they may not suit everyone's personal requirements.

- Rice cooker — very easy to use and clean, you don't have to worry about boiling water, or timing.
- Turbo cooker with timer — does a variety of cooking tasks.
- Silicon baking mats — for placing inside trays, to stop sticking and make removing items easier.
- George Foreman frypan/cooker — many say this is easy to use and clean.
- Tupperware measuring cups and spoons — come in different shapes and colours, you don't have to see to use them.
- Induction ovens and hot plates — have easy-to-use hot plates that are very safe for people who are blind as they are instantly cool when lifting the pot off, although special pots are required.
- Thermomix processor and oven. — contact Thermomix for sales of older tactile versions.
- Pen Friend — digital organiser.
- Bessemer pots — heavy and stable; highly regarded for their excellent heat transfer.
- MasterChef Mezzaluna Chopper & Board set — http://www.yourhomedepot.com.au/masterchef-443-mezzaluna-chopper-board-set-na.html; buy online.
- Boil Alert (or Milk Saver) — warns you when a liquid is beginning to boil.

- Talking thermometers — for personal (health) use, as well as use in the kitchen.
- Baseball cap with an LED light under peak.
- Bat Lights — spotlights that are useful in the kitchen.
- Butcher's Gloves — protective mesh gloves for use with sharp knives.
- Portable lights — for above the kitchen bench or in the pantry.
- Mandala cutting device — to make slicing vegetables easier.
- Timer with bell alarm (mechanical or electronic) or use smartphone — recommended when poor vision prevents you seeing a clock.
- Cutting knives with saw-like handles — can be useful when you have arthritis or weak wrists.
- Slow cookers — recommended for ease of use, but good organisation is required for keeping recepies and preparation of ingredients.
- Liquid level sensors — to place on cups when pouring liquids; they give an alert at two stages.
- As pouring liquids are usually difficult with low vision, a Left-hand soup ladle might assist.
- Talking scales — useful for kitchen or bathroom.
- Talking liquid measuring jug.
- Remember, use tactile markers as a low cost option.

Reference Books

In addition to Google and other voice recognition devices, some audio Reference Books available from blind agencies include:

- Kitchen — Nigella Lawson

- The 1,000 Recipe Cookbook — Martha Day
- Cooking For VIP — Maxine Turkett
- The Margaret Fulton Cookbook
- Four ingredients Cookbook
- Scales Away — BCA's cookbook — over 600 easy recipes

17

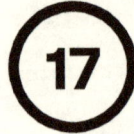

Orientation and Mobility, Dogs versus Canes, Safety and Travel

'I kept wondering when this mobility and orientation course would end. Then it would hit me, the course would never end. This was my life!'

Dr Jane Poulson

'I do not think, sir, you have any right to command me, merely because you are older than I, or because you have seen more of the world than I have; your claim to superiority depends on the use you have made of your time and experience.'

Charlotte Brontë, Jane Eyre

Once More, it's All about Skills and Attitude

My personal reluctance to use a white cane and receive training in the early days of my vision loss was echoed time and time again by the experience of peers who had already adjusted to sight loss. One peer in particular, Leanne from Victoria, said it best. 'Of all the supports I've received, I think Orientation and Mobility support is the most important! It gives me the confidence to get to work and get out and about again!'

Yet, of all the symbols of blindness, the white cane is perhaps the most feared, the most vilified, for it represents the shame of blindness. Why? It all seems so contradictory. Perhaps the response of Dr Jane Poulson of Canada, who describes the feelings of resentment before accepting blindness, said it well. 'I loathed each new thing I had to learn how to do ... I wanted to strangle the instructors who were congratulating me on making it down a set of stairs safely. Nothing could break through the thick layer of anger, fear, loathing and resentment that enveloped me during those dreadful days.'[189]

As I have described in earlier chapters, you don't have to be 'black' blind to use a cane or a dog guide. Many people using the white cane still have useable sight as do dog guide users. The white cane is an important navigational tool and guide, yet nearly all clients I met were reluctant to use a white cane. I shared these feelings, and it wasn't until my son purchased a white cane for me that I reluctantly changed my view.

The Role of Orientation and Mobility Specialists

As our vision is lost or decreases, one of the principal skills to learn is how to get out and about safely. We call this mobility. As we navigate our diminished environment successfully, we call this orientation. Thus the specially trained support workers who help us succeed in this area are called Orientation and Mobility (O&M) specialists. They undertake a two-year course designed to understand a client's needs, their psyche in confronting vision loss and how clients must re-skill themselves to use their other senses in order to travel safely.

Many people when first experiencing vision loss are reluctant to use an O&M specialists. Again much of this reluctance is based on feelings that we are not yet ready for such instruction; fear of what others might say and resistance to change. To quote Dr. Jane Poulson again, she describes feelings of someone approaching mobility training: 'I wanted to walk in a straight line, upstairs, use the escalator, walk through a revolving door, to get onto the correct elevator when the bell rang, walk on the sidewalks even if the pavement was cracked, to avoid falling into manholes, to walk in the park in the sunlight, hear the birds singing and children playing ... note the traffic sounds to figure out my position. I did not want to experience something as basic as walking, as a terror filled, monumental challenge. I wanted pleasure and relaxation from walking. I wanted independent mobility and a mind free to wander and enjoy as I want. I was determined to achieve this.'[190]

The apprehension expressed by Jane Poulson can be quite legitimate as people feel at the beginning of vision loss they do not actually need this service, or that they need a cane. 'Oh, my eyes are OK, I can still see where I'm going!' is a typical stoic response heard in my discussion groups. Nevertheless, learning key skills at an early stage is a great confidence booster, as well as allowing you to go out safely.

A key proposition of this book is that we are all individuals, our vision loss varies significantly between everyone and there is no one-size-fits-all approach. Understanding what a client can or cannot see is important. Many with vision loss will experience loss of night vision, or experience severe glare during the day, limiting capacity and increasing risk of injury. However, the key factors that need to be considered by an individual are:

- What is your degree of vision loss? Can I see steps, bollards, obstacles clearly?
- Am I likely to fall, or have already tripped over?
- Can I see well at night time? Or in going from a bright street into a dark shop, or vice versa, do I feel I can't see?
- Can I walk around safely? Am I bumping into furniture, other people, or glass doors?
- Am I avoiding going out because I feel nervous?
- In using public transport do I feel apprehensive?
- Am I walking with poor posture, with my head bent down in order that I can see the pavement?

The above factors are some of the many reasons why an O&M specialist can help.

The response of those who do use a cane is, as Julia from New

South Wales said, 'My life changed positively once I began using a cane and I found so many strangers want to help me!'

As we move from full to restricted sight, we may not be using our remaining sight effectively (see Chapter 9 on how to use remaining sight), along with our other senses such as touch, hearing and smell to assist our progress. There is much to be learnt. For example, how our environment varies, using any remaining sight to assist with orientation, watching out for landmarks and familiar settings.

What Do Orientation and Mobility Specialists Do?

O&M specialists train you to have the skills and confidence that help you in the home, in getting to work, orientating yourself around large shopping centres, using escalators, travelators and lifts, managing large open spaces, and learning how to avoid becoming disorientated or lost. They will also train you to use public transport, and in the use of mobility aids and GPS technology.

Importantly, they will also speak to and educate your family on the impacts of low vision and on sighted guide techniques — see below.

One dominant fear often articulated is that 'An O&M will make me use a cane!' That is absolutely not true, there is no compulsion. The cane is seen as a symbol of blindness, yet it remains a vital navigational tool. It is a matter of knowledge of how a cane might help and to trust it. A white cane conveniently folds up, and it is better to carry it with you to deal with problematic situations — like crossing a busy road, or finding yourself in an unfamiliar or dark environment — than not to have one.

An O&M specialist will explain how to use a cane, how it can help, and then allow you to trial a cane to see how you feel about it. It is a discreet, private and respectful service. If you feel embarrassed about practising how to use a white cane near your home, they will take you to an unfamiliar area.

O&Ms will also teach you how to use your other faculties to greater advantage. For example, when you are walking, to feel changes in pavement surfaces, how to improve your orientation by using landmarks such as shops, fences, trees, and the sounds of, say, schools or traffic, and if you have remaining sight, how to identify major buildings or other landmarks. They also train you to use smell as a key skill for orientation — smells of a chemist, baker, butcher, coffee shop, op shops all have distinct differences. Some people with vision impairment do report issues with hearing, smell and touch, so in these circumstances a different training program is prepared.

Many clients reported that to cross a road, they would 'rely upon hearing and that large arterial roads were difficult to cross where no pedestrian traffic lights exist'. This dare-Devil practice is extremely dangerous. A driver cannot tell you have limited sight and relies upon you to also keep a lookout. Many people reported 'near misses' and other instances, 'where a courteous driver might stop and wave, but this was of little value when you could not see the driver, nor the car speeding alongside in a second outer lane'. O&Ms will spend much time on identifying where best places are located for crossing roads and how to cross a road safely. In short, O&Ms enable us to overcome many of the day-to-day fears and barriers we encounter in getting out and about with vision loss.

O&Ms also act as personal advocates with local authorities

if changes such as fixing dangerous pavement or installing pedestrian crossings or lights are needed. Local councils also respond well to such requests knowing they are prepared by a professional.

Key skills offered by an O&M include, how to navigate and use public transport, and how to ask for and obtain help in the form required (See 'Asking For Help and Sighted Guide Techniques', below.) An O&M will also provide as much training as you need — there is no one attempt and that's all!

Many people use an O&M support even with a dog guide when they need to go to new areas or locations. As Susie Barrington from Sydney says, 'Orientation is an ongoing, constant process!' That is a view supported by Dr Jane Poulson, who said, 'I learnt to navigate the region ... by listening to clues like one way traffic, or certain smells like the Body Shop ... I learned to rely upon fixed landmarks.'[191]

Blindness support Agencies in Australia and overseas provide O&M specialists. Apart from your personal training, an O&M specialist can also discuss vision loss and 'acceptance' issues with your work, school or members of your family. Understanding by others that you need a cane and why, is just as important for your success. As earlier mentioned, there are many examples of partners, parents or children resisting the taking up of a cane because they are embarrassed by it, and don't want to see a family member as disabled. We expect our family to understand us, but we need to become educators.

Getting Used to the White Cane

The white cane, or 'long cane' as it is also known, is recognised everywhere as a symbol of blindness. But, as mentioned, it also seems to symbolise the stigma of blindness more than any other object.

In the confidence of group discussions where partners are usually excluded to encourage openness, clients reported that husbands and children are reluctant to have mother use a cane. Families are also reluctant to learn Sighted Guide techniques so that safety is maintained. A woman about to take a trip to Brisbane with her family, reported that they were 'all supporting me', but still didn't like her using a white cane. I asked her, 'How did you get along and how does your family help in a strange city?' She said, 'Oh, I walk by myself and just put my hand out and follow the walls of buildings!'

Yet it has to be remembered before rushing to judgement, that sighted family members may also be grieving over sight loss of a family member and feel awkward in raising the subject, or being associated with the stigma. If the person with vision loss is reluctant, or has difficulty talking about how their vision loss affects them, or is tired of trying to explain it, then a communication gap will remain. Getting an O&M specialist to talk to the whole family will help.

If you are partially sighted, here are some common responses:

The first thoughts are ones of denial, for example thoughts like, 'I don't want to use it,' 'I'll be fine without it,' 'Holding a cane stresses me,' 'White canes and sun glasses are not for me,' 'What if my friends see me with it, they'll say I'm really blind now!' Anxious thoughts are naturally part of our acceptance pathway.[192]

Barbara Pierce, noted social commentator in the US, says on canes, 'If a blind person begins early to use a white cane and gets really good at it, he/she will feel more comfortable being watched. Most of us feel less at ease under observation when we expect to make mistakes. Good cane users do not necessarily do everything right, but they can move smoothly and with confidence. Ultimately, perfection is not the object. The point is to get safely and independently where one wants to go.'

Barbara deals with one of the most vexing issues for those with vision impairment: how to navigate a crowd and break into groups. She says, 'One thing to be said about a really long white cane is that it is not easily overlooked, and it certainly explains why its user slips into a group saying brightly, "And who is here?" I picked my group carefully, avoiding the ones deeply engrossed in conversation. I would slide between groups until I heard a familiar voice or found a group engaged in superficial chat. I might overhear a question that I could answer, and I would insert myself into a group that way.'[193]

When you are not prepared to use a cane and still in early stages of adjustment to vision loss, socialising in large groups can present some difficulties. Professor Emeritus, David Macmillan from Victoria, a blind vision-support group leader, confirms a common experience for the vision impaired. Joining a large gathering of people presents great difficulties, particularly if many are not known. At a conference, for instance, how do you determine who is there? How do you enter and engage with those present without drawing attention and disrupting conversations. How do you find particular persons with whom you wish to speak? He recommends a technique he calls 'Trapezing'. Enter the gathering with a trusted friend or work colleague who is familiar with the crowd. He/she is your first spotter, introducing you to the first person you want to meet. When you are done with the person on that trapeze, ask him to swing you across to the next person or a new spotter. Alternatively, you can ask a spotter to watch for when a target person is free to talk, and then to swing you over. In this way you can swing around and work the room. David adds, 'Trapezing is efficient and reduces stress. It really works'. I can vouch for this method. It reinforces the principle, when you can no longer see things, rely upon another person to help. As CEO, I did similar using Board Members to identify and connect with people I needed to meet.

Another typical problem at social groups is that, often the well-meaning hostess will say, 'Oh, welcome, come over here and sit down!' This approach is expressed so often so as to make one think that people with vision impairment are particularly fatigued or frail. Do hosts or hostesses say this to all guests? Perhaps they do, but such custom can leave you stranded, stuck in a chair in the corner of a room. While seated, you are not at speaking level and, unless someone knows you and picks you up, your evening can be isolated and socially deadly. Try to stand in a good location if that's what is happening, it gives you a better opportunity to circulate if that is what you prefer. Alternatively, rely upon a friend to be your social guide.

Dining out at large eight- or ten-seat round tables can also make it difficult for a person with vision impairment to function when so much conversation on these large tables depends on eye contact to engage and even lip reading if the locale is noisy. Generally speaking, square or rectangular tables give you more scope to converse. By sitting at a corner, you can talk to at least two people on each side.

The vast majority of vision impaired people in discussion groups have said something like, 'I was given a cane but it remained folded up in my cupboard for months!' We feel embarrassed or vulnerable in using it. A young lady with low vision wrote in the Blind Alliance Newsletter, 2019, 'I always try my best to dodge the obstacles around me using my low vision. Sometimes my best doesn't quite cut it. People and objects appear out of the blurry fog (i.e. my vision) too quickly for me to react and get out of the way. These days, people are busy on their phones, rude, and nobody has time to watch out for a blind girl! Especially if they can't tell that I'm blind! Situations can get stressful for me and for the friends or family who are trying to guide me. It took me months to realize that using a cane would remedy some of these stressful times.'[194]

Using a White Cane in Crowds

A considerable number of people using a cane have difficulty in crowded places. A person said one day in a group discussion, 'I'm worried about being in crowds and inadvertently tapping the ankles of others with my cane.' An O&M specialist who happened to be at this meeting said, 'Well, you know, this is your right! Your right by tapping others gently lets others know that you can't see them. It is they, the public, who must look out for you!' Now, isn't that the correct perspective? Yes! Of course it is! But if you are recently experiencing vision impairment, and still coming to terms with your situation and the increased assertiveness required, it is hard to accept these different rules.

In today's environment, many, many people are walking around using smartphones or texting and are not concentrating on their surroundings. Once members of the public realise you are using a cane, they apologise to you for 'blocking' your way. So they should;

it is they who have the responsibility to look out. Don't expect to be the one responsible for crowd navigation.

More on Canes

Sighted people often think that a person using a cane can't see at all, and they often overreact. This can be upsetting to some and lead to unwanted offers of assistance. As one person with vision impairment at a discussion group said, 'I am a person with restricted vision and resisted using a cane for many years until my son, witnessing this display of stubborn stupidity, bought me one! It was the very best thing I have done!'

As mentioned earlier, admitting publicly that you have vision loss and a disability, is a great emotional struggle. This is largely because blindness has been imposed upon us without choice and our fear of disclosure has a disempowering impact. However, once this issue of embarrassment is dealt with, a cane provides the following benefits:

- It acts like an extension to your hand/finger to reach down to ground level and feel for pavement unevenness, gutters, steps and obstacles and prevents falls.
- The cane tells other people that you have poor vision and that they should make allowances for this.
- The cane gives you back control over your environment, helps measure width and depth of gutters, stairs, or the step when disembarking transport.

- It reverses an onus of proof where others are about to blame you for bumping into them; they soon apologise and cannot do enough to help.
- It warns public transport operators to 'look out' for you, to advise when your stop is coming up, and warns drivers that they must take care.

Types of Cane

The O&M specialist will show you the many different types of canes and work out with you which one is best. Some types of canes are:

- a short ID cane usually held across your front at an angle but not touching the ground — it is just to tell others you have vision issues
- a long white cane that comes up to your sternum or higher and which you hold in one hand with the tip touching the ground
- a lightweight fibreglass long cane for people with weak wrists or arthritis
- a short white but strong support cane with a handle for balance.

All of the above are collapsible and can fold up into your bag or backpack. This makes them ideal to carry with you just in case you might need a cane. When you find yourself crossing a street, or catching a bus, or in a disorientating place, you can bring out your cane.

Canes can have different tips to suit conditions such as rough pavements and grass surfaces, including:

- golf ball or tennis ball size rolling tips, which move across from side to side
- a pear-shaped tip for tapping the ground as well as sideways movement
- a jumbo roller for very rough surfaces or sand
- a 'Bindu Basher', like a large hook, for rough paths or bush walking.

Dog versus Cane

Susie Barrington from Sydney, who is totally blind, tells of how, 'One day when in a bank, my dog guide Haly had taken me up to the counter, but I couldn't see and didn't realise I was actually there. I said, Haly, 'find the counter, Find the counter! But, she couldn't, she was already there! Frustrated with this command, Haly jumped up on top of the counter!' How smart is that? Perhaps Susie should have opened up a bank account for her dog straight away with a big performance bonus?

A dog guide can be clever, funny, smart and sneaky — always looking for that extra snack! But a more loving, caring and protective companion cannot be found.

But as Erik Weihenmayer, totally blind adventurer, admitted, 'Working with a dog guide was harder than I thought.' The process involved a lot of trial and error. Find the stairs, escalator, chair, etc. His dog guide, 'Wizard' an Alsatian, even picked up spare change he had dropped, 'handing it to me all slobbery and wet'. (Note: most dog guides don't pick up change!)

Unfortunately, a number of dog guide users report being denied access to taxis, restaurants and other venues. This type of discrimination is also reported to take place in other countries. In some instances, taxi drivers with certain cultural beliefs, refuse to pick up a person with their dog guide. This is illegal and penalties apply. Dog guide users and their dogs are protected in Australia by the Commonwealth Disability Discrimination Act (DDA) 1992,:'9 (2) For the purposes of this Act, an assistance animal is a dog or other animal: — accredited under a law of a State or Territory that provides for the accreditation of animals trained to assist a persons with a disability to alleviate the effect of the disability...'

All Australian states have supporting Protection of Domestic Animals Acts with penalties applying if dog guides are not allowed into most premises. The exceptions usually are — certain zoos, hospital operating theatres, commercial kitchens and hospital burns units. Dog guides are allowed in Intensive Care Units, restaurants and dental clinics, among other areas.

A dog guide is a personal choice and there are many practical reasons supporting this. Some people are allergic to dogs or dog hair, some do not want the obligation of maintaining a dog. A common complaint with blonde Labradors is that their hair can be seen on everything. Dog guide providers insist that cane training be undertaken first, because, for example, there might be times when your dog might not be able to work. It could be too hot or the dog may be sick, etc.

In a recent group discussion, a participant, Maria from Queensland said, 'I just started using my cane, I was very scared and on entering a railway station, a group of young people ran up the ramp in a hurry knocking me over. I think I should get a dog; it will be safer!' However, the group's vision impaired and highly trained peer, Leanne, a dog guide user of over 20 years advised,

'Having a dog guide doesn't guarantee safety in a crowd.' On a dog guide's capacity to keep you safe, Leanne said, 'I have fallen when tripping over a raised footpath tile of only a few centimetres. The dog doesn't tell you this by its movements as they are too slight!' This view is supported by Susie Barrington, who says, 'There is not much tactile feedback with a dog but it allows freedom of movement where you are free to stand up straight and allow your other senses to work for you. The dog's role is to see the barriers and take you safely around them. In crossing a street, the dog will stop at the pavement's edge. It is not the dog's role to see the cars; you must make the decision to cross!'

The best tactic to adopt in crowds is to stop and wait from them to pass or in a moment like Maria experienced, stop and if possible move to the side. This practice is also helpful when using escalators. In a dense crowd, people may not see your dog or cane.

In order that you can keep your composure in these situations, also allow yourself more time so that you are not also panic stricken, rushing to catch the next train. There will always be another service coming!

To many, a dog guide is more acceptable than a cane. A dog is usually much admired and attracts people to come and speak to it, rather than you. People will come up and want to talk to a dog guide and often say, 'How beautiful and clever it is! Does it really understand what you are saying?' Owners are always required to ask people not to touch a dog guide when in harness as this distracts the dog from concentrating.

Dog guides are trained to take you on trips they have been trained to make, such as shopping, work, travel or school. They are also trained to find pedestrian crossing light buttons and office counters, to stop at stairs and make sure you are at the hand rail, to guide you to a train carriage or bus door and a seat, then patiently place themselves under the seat. The concentration required of the dog explains why, when in harness, a dog guide should not be talked to or played with. Their amazing concentration will be broken.

Dog guides are trained to usually walk on the left of a person, and are trained to keep an eye on their owner's right shoulder to protect against collisions. They avoid obstacles and stop at kerbs. They know their left from their right. A dog can understand as many as 200 words. Sometimes dogs might lead their owner into overhanging branches because it is trickier for them to judge overhead obstacles. It all takes practice. It's a partnership, and owners often consider they are driving the dog rather than being led by it.

Naturally, not all dogs succeed in becoming guides; temperament is all-important. Dog guide users also have to be trained in handling dogs. Some behavioural issues arise when the owner does not follow dog management principles. A dog sees itself as part of a 'pack' and you, not it, must be 'top dog'!

At between 10 and 11 years dog guides mostly retire after eight to nine years of service. A dog guide may become noticeably 'mentally fatigued' after so many years of training and concentration on guiding, but it is often arthritis which ends a dog's working life. When a dog retires, the owner can experience significant grief and sadness at the loss of such a friend and companion. A home is usually found for its retirement if keeping two dogs is not possible.

In considering a dog guide, you must have sound reasons to need one, such as lots of travel or work. Dog guides are not social 'companion' dogs, they are working dogs and cost approximately $A50,000 each to breed and train, plus an additional A$30,000 for associated training with its new owner. These costs are currently being paid by NDIS in Australia.

If you feel you need a dog guide, your needs will be assessed, and a dog is matched both to your needs and personality. As there is a waiting list, it is best to go on all lists. In Australia, the two dog guide providers are Vision Australia's Seeing Eye Dogs (SED) and the Guide Dogs Associations in most states.

There is, however, a responsibility to look after, feed, groom and walk a dog, but as most cane users say, 'A cane requires none of this, you just put it in the corner when you get home!'

On the plus side, a dog guide is a good 'ice breaker', although the dog might be the centre of attention.Graeme Innes took some umbrage over the fact that people will more willingly talk to a dog guide rather than its handler, but this only confirms points made earlier in this book, that people are unsure, or afraid of what to ask or say to people who are blind. Perhaps the reality is that domesticated dogs play an unusually close role with mankind and are normally a centre of attraction. Mark Twain said of dogs, 'When you go to Heaven, leave your dog outside. Entry into Heaven is by way of favour, not merit. If it was the latter and you took in your dog, you might find yourself left outside and the dog taken in!'

Getting Out and About

Venturing out into the wider world can be made much less intimidating with the right planning, knowledge of help at hand,

and a confident approach. Remember: be assertive; it is your right to be treated as well as any other and to get more help if you need it.

If you are going out to the movies or the theatre, use Audio Description. A Companion Card in Australia allows you to bring along a friend, who gets in free of charge.

Download all travel apps. (See Chapter 18, Technology and Working in the Shed.) If you don't know how to download them, get a friend to help you.

If using taxis, have a clear plan so that you can give the driver directions. Ask drivers to assist you by, for example, taking you to the shop or airport door. Yes, that is part of their job. On the financial side, apply for a Taxi Subsidy.

Use your mobile phone to ring the shop, or with a medical appointment, ring the office and ask for someone to come out and meet you. Yes, they will do this, but you need to remain courteous! Of course, you must be organised so that the phone number is in your phone. Also, use virtual assistants such as Apple's Siri to ask, 'Where am I?' to tell you where you are, or use GPS systems.

Ask the shop attendant to help you. Ask members of the public to assist. Most people like helping you and this actually increases your independence, not lessens it. It works!

Be aware of tactile tiles. Many sighted people do not know the purpose of these aids, which are often placed on a footpath, the edge of a train platform, or along other pedestrian areas. There are two styles. One, a long series of raised parallel strips to indicate direction, and the second, a series of raised squares or circles which provide a warning that you have reached the edge of a road or train platform and to stop. They are usually yellow or red/orange in colour.

Safety and Fears of Vulnerability

As earlier mentioned, a common reason for not using a white cane is a fear that this will 'make me more vulnerable to be attacked and robbed'. Let us briefly review the general state of assault and violence in Australia, England and the USA.

As identified by the Australian Bureau of Statistics, while there is growing awareness within Australia of increased family violence, there is little or nothing pertaining to people with vision loss. In summary, 'Intimate partner violence causes more assaults. Women are at greater risk of family, domestic and sexual violence. Men are more likely to experience violence from strangers and in a public place; women are most likely to know the perpetrator (often their current or a previous partner) and the violence usually takes place in their home. Between 2005 and 2016, rates of partner violence against women have remained relatively stable.'[195]

NOTE: More recent information arising from domestic violence data suggests a significant increase in reported cases. So, violence is more likely at home than elsewhere, and for those worried about blindness making them more vulnerable, especially once they commence using a cane, there is little evidence in Australia, England, the USA or Europe that using a cane heightens vulnerability in the community. Confidence in walking to your destination is important to deter the opportunistic thief.

However, looking at vulnerability in the disability sector broadly, it is understandable that people, especially older people, with a disability may be apprehensive. According to the Australian Network on Disability, 'Generally, 50.7% of those 65 years and over have a disability, compared to 12.5% under 65years. 35.9% of households have a person with a disability. Most people with disabilities (87 per cent) are restricted in carrying out at least one everyday activity, such as self-care, mobility or communication.'[196]

'Research has shown that more than a quarter of people who report sexual assault have a disability. 90 per cent of women with intellectual disabilities have been sexually abused but from someone who is known to them.'[197]

Statistics from the USA also indicate a higher vulnerability for those with a disability generally compared to the public. Data indicates a rate of 12.7 disabled people per 1,000 as compared to3.9 ordinary people, are victims of assault or crimes. But this is disability generally. There is little or no evidence of assault or violence against those with vision disability.

It appears younger people are more vulnerable than those aged 65 and older. However, those with cognitive disabilities had a significantly higher rate — 56.6 per 1,000. Disturbingly, as mentioned above, higher rates (40 per cent) were committed by people who knew the victim.[198]

Statistics specifically identifying a risk for vision impaired people do not appear to be available in Australia, or for that matter, other countries. The Australian Human Rights Commission states, 'Although much is known about many aspects of family, domestic and sexual violence, there are several data gaps that need to be filled to present a comprehensive picture of its extent and impact in Australia. Specifically, there is no, or limited, data on: children, indigenous and those with disability.'[199]

O&Ms with many years of experience in mobility instruction regularly report that, 'Using a cane enables you to walk with greater confidence and this fact makes yourself less vulnerable.' People with low vision tend to peer at the ground and stoop. A cane allows you to walk in an upright posture, not be hesitant or slow, and to move confidently. The confidence in moving surely and quickly from place to place makes you less vulnerable as it provides less chance for an opportunist thief.

Using Public Transport

Many people when first told they have to give up driving may have never used public transport before. Indeed the very thought of using it can create significant anxiety. With vision loss, the main problems are identifying route numbers, knowing schedule times, flagging down the correct bus or tram, knowing routes, finding a seat or having the confidence to ask for one, knowing where to disembark, entry and exit onto unfamiliar pavement, and fears of other traffic.

If you are threatened, alert transport staff or other passengers. Call the police. Have the number on your phone so you can just ask Siri or Google voice to ring the emergency number (000 in Australia).

Preparation

Plan your journey, try to minimise waiting times by using a journey planner on your GPS, or public transport app. You might need training to use the app first.

Make sure you can be seen, choose well-lit paths if possible, stand where you can be seen. If you are totally blind, working with an O&M specialist will identify these safe areas.

If a person is standing too close to you on public transport, move your bag to the front of you and turn to face them.

Take the time, or use an O&M specialist to train you, to locate safety features like emergency buttons, CCTV cameras; as mentioned earlier, use the program called AIRA Vision if possible as you will get real time human guidance.

Keep valuables concealed, bags secured.

Be ready with your door keys and don't fumble; if possible, use external motion light sensors. Many vision impaired people say that placing their key in the door is difficult and struggle to 'see' where to place the key. Remember, break the habit of trying to see, you don't need to, using touch is much easier; have your important keys marked.

Police advise, Resist someone trying to get you to move elsewhere on a train, tram or a bus; these cases have 80 per cent negative outcomes.[200]

In addition to mobility training, skills and confidence in handling money reduce the likelihood of being taken advantage of. For example, as mentioned earlier in Chapter 16, having a clear system for organisation of bank notes in your wallet or purse as well as using a coin holder can lessen vulnerability. (See Chapter 16, Independence in the Home, Community and Kitchen.)

Transport for the disability sector generally creates problems. 'Despite progress towards making all public transport in Australia fully accessible by 2022, 1.2 million people with disabilities report difficulties using public transport.'[201]

An O&M specialist can assist you by going with you and training you in skills that include catching a bus, tram or train, managing crowds, managing lifts and escalators, how to travel safely and access seating, how to identify the bus you want and stop it. Some tips here are: To hold up a large laminated card for the bus driver to see with your required bus number, although this is where a folding cane is more practical and public transport drivers or conductors are trained to understand what a white cane means and assist you. If you hold out your cane, a bus will pull over for you. If it is not the right bus, this doesn't matter; it is their duty to stop. Most probably the driver will tell you when your bus is coming.

Many people using Wheelie Walkers or electric chairs cannot hold a cane. But they find by just taping a cane on their walker or chair so that it is visible will get the idea across to others that the user cannot see very well. Alternatively, make a large A4 laminated sign saying 'I've got low vision', and tape it onto your walker or chair.

GPS public transport apps are free and work well with built-in audio software on smartphones. They will give you information on bus, tram or train schedules, and this will help you flag down the correct bus or tram.

In railway stations or on trains, staff and drivers will 'look out' for you and provide assistance.

Asking For Help, and Sighted Guide Techniques

As mentioned, getting out and about presents us with some of our greatest challenges. Fear and hyperventilating occur when we become stressed, and we may need to stop and take deep breaths to settle us down before we can ask directions. Often in these situations we have to stop a stranger and ask for help. Although many people may pass you by, what often happens is that a willing helper may grab you by the arm or hand, then push you ahead of them to cross a road or enter a building. Apart from bringing you into unwanted proximity to a stranger, grabbing your arm is unhelpful, because doing so places you ahead, slightly in front of the other person and they may not then tell you where a step is or whether it is up or down. It is usually quite frightening to feel 'pushed'.

The most successful form of guidance by another person is what we call the sighted guide technique. The basic technique is where you, the vision impaired person, lightly hold the elbow or shoulder of the person guiding, which places you half a body width, or approximately one half step, behind, but you still remain to their side walking comfortably. In this position you can follow them and it is amazing how much information you can get from the other person by just lightly holding them with thumb and finger. If they move sideways, up, down or veer, you can feel this movement and follow. If you get apprehensive, you can easily let go and stop. If you are a cane user, it is still best to carry it as this warns those coming towards you that one has a vision problem and it is they who should make space.

If a 'sighted guide' is properly trained as a family member or friend might be, they will also warn you of bollards and narrow spaces (as in restaurants), tell you if stairs are 'up or down' and take you to a handrail for further support.

On approaching narrow access ways, they will move their arm

with you, still holding on, behind their back and you can then move behind them to follow in single file. In exiting the narrow space, they move their arm back to their side and you can then walk as a pair again.

In coming to a chair, it is best for the sighted guide to take your hand and place it on top of the back of a chair, then leave you to feel your way to sit down. This method is easier than trying to get you to sit down, it leaves you in control and you can take your own time. Finding a table is similar: place the back of the hand lower than table height. This avoids touching hot surfaces and knocking over items.

A good sighted guide will also not say 'over there' when giving directions, but give the clock method and distances.

A key aspect of the sighted guide technique is that they give you back control over your environment. They are empowering, a major factor improving our capacity to be assertive and independent. For example, if a stranger or friend grabs our arm and starts pushing us, we can say, 'Stop! Do you mind, I'd like to hold your elbow please!' You might need to explain briefly why this is so and which side you prefer, but as you can let go at any time if apprehensive, you are in control of your space, not the guide. This technique also allows for body space, where you are not drawn in too close to a stranger.

Local and Overseas Travel: Assistance

As already noted, many people in early stages of vision loss find using public transport systems confronting. Many, having driven cars all their lives, will not have previously used public transport, and therefore be apprehensive. Like all re-skilling, it is a matter of knowing how the system works. The following summary offers some tips.

Some travel assistance supports in Australia include:

- A Disability Pension — Blind: this pension offers concessions which allow free transport on all Metropolitan Government services, with discounts for country travel.
- The Companion Card already referred to, allows a companion to travel free of charge with you.
- Vision Impaired Travel Pass this is provided by state transport authorities. In all states, if you are Legally Blind or have total vision loss, you receive free transport on trains, trams, buses (including some private), urban and inter urban. Contact your state transport authority for more information. Great Southern Railway; Indian Pacific, Overlander and Ghan have generous concessions.

Transport Mobility Allowance

If you are working, volunteering for more than 15 hours per week, or studying, the Mobility Allowance is available, up to A$139 per fortnight. (Note: Now subsumed within NDIS.)

This allowance is provided by the Commonwealth Department of Human Services (DHS): https://www.humanservices.gov.au/customer/services/centrelink/mobility-allowance

To qualify, you must:

- be 16 years of age or older
- meet residency requirements

- be unable to use public transport without substantial assistance because of disability, illness, or injury
- provide a medical report from your doctor confirming you cannot use public transport
- travel to and from home for paid work, voluntary work, study or training, or to look for work.

If there is no public transport where you live, you may still be eligible for the Mobility Allowance. Voluntary work must be for a charitable, welfare or community organisation. Study or training can include secondary school, tertiary studies, trade and vocational courses. This benefit is income and asset test free non-taxable and reportable for tax.

Travel Assistance Overseas

Generally speaking, travelling overseas will test your capacity to be pleasantly 'assertive'. Knowing your benefits and in some cases rights is a good start. In some cases, playing 'the blind person' is necessary. Therefore wearing an ID badge or using a white cane makes a world of difference when approaching staff members at train stations or airports. Always carry a folding cane with you!

Safety issues are of course always present, so use the well-developed Meet and Assist program (see below), or train disability services. (Adopt careful practices of handling money as detailed in Chapter16.)

Money is always a concern, but banks have a special cash card for overseas money which offer high security as long as you know your password. However, you can only draw down funds from an ATM, not across the counter. Otherwise, get a money belt.

There are many pickpockets overseas and they are highly skilled. Don't leave valuables in a visible position, don't put all your money in one place, and be aware that even leather bags can be cut open without you noticing it by skilled pickpockets. You can purchase protective covers for passports, credit cards and cash cards which prevent scanning by hidden devices or highly skilled operators. Dense crowds are always a high risk for having your pockets or bags picked. Have a special system for organising your money before you go out.

An amusing story highlights this point. A friend told of how, while navigating a dense crowd on a busy railway station, she thought little of receiving a few bumps. Happily seated in her carriage and looking onto the platform, a grinning man held up her passport for her to see as the train moved off.

If you are travelling in Europe, public transport disability assistance is available in most countries. Preferably reserve this service at least five days prior to travel. The service is very good and will take you to the platform, wait until the train comes, get you on board and to your seat. This is most helpful as European trains are very long and your seat (if reserved) may be a long way down a crowded platform. You need to be in the proximate location of the right wagon to avoid high stress. Likewise, if reserving and travelling in an overnight sleeper wagon, the service is excellent.

Meet and Assist

This service supports your airline travel within Australia and overseas. You must reserve this service when booking your ticket. When you register at the reception desk, someone with the service takes you through security and Customs, if travelling overseas, and takes you to your departure lounge. On arriving, a person will meet you, take you through the arrivals process, help find your luggage and take you to your next on-service. Often they will place you in a wheelchair, but don't worry, while this might initially appear patronizing and confronting, it is actually quite efficient. This wonderful service makes independent travel possible.

Note: There is a private Meet and Assist, which charges to assist people through terminals. Do not confused this service with the Disability Meet and Assist, which is free. Some travel agents don't know of Meet and Assist, so be prepared.

If you're intending to fly, while you might prefer a window seat, ask for an aisle seat when booking your ticket as aircrew are more able to assist you and you can identify when they are near.

Australian Restrictions on Pension Travel

Currently the time allowed for travel outside Australia for Disability Support Pensions (DSP) is four weeks. If you exceed this time your DSP will be cancelled. However, for the DSP — Blind, important exemptions apply:

1. You must contact Centrelink and inquire if your DSP — Blind is classified as Manifest. Manifest means permanent disability — the test is Legally Blind or worse.
2. If your Centrelink file is classified as 'Manifest', portability of travel conditions will automatically apply, allowing limited travel of up to 25 weeks to cover short-term overseas trips.

3. You must ascertain whether your file is marked as 'Manifest.' Call the International Section of Centrelink on: 131 673.

4. If you stay overseas for longer than four weeks, some side benefits — for example, Mobility Allowance, phone and energy supplements — will be suspended but reinstated upon your return.

In reviewing your file, Centrelink may ask you for an updated medical report, but this will depend on their subsequent assessment confirming you are 'manifestly' blind — meaning permanent.

(18)

Technology and Working in the Shed

'Information and ignorance are like light and darkness
... When light comes into your room, darkness must fly
away. When information rules your mind, ignorance
finds its way out!'

Israel More Ayivor, The Great Hand Book of Quotes

'Don't let the noise of others' opinions drown out your
own inner voice.'

*Steve Jobs, Stanford University commencement
speech, 2005*

What Technology Is Best

As has often been discussed in this book, after many years
of sight, one of the hardest changes we face is to break the

habit of wanting to look at everything. It is our first and most powerful natural sensory instinct. As a result we continue to 'blindly' struggle on, unless we know and accept there are better alternative ways of processing information, the 'noise of other's opinions' as Steve Jobs would say.

Current technology is now truly fantastic! As stated throughout this book, the great message is that with text-to-speech audio function, you do not have to see it to use it. With voice recognition devices, access is even easier.

At the outset, there is one particular point that needs clarifying. Many sighted people know about and suggest that with smartphones, vision impaired people need only use Siri in iPhones, or Ask Google in Androids. This is only half the story. You can use these voice recognition features for opening up apps on the phone, making reminders, and so on. However, text-to-speech features are what make these phones and tablets fantastic for those with vision loss. But first, the text-to-speech functions in smartphones must be turned on. They are:

- in all Apple products Voice Over
- in Samsung Android Talk Back.

These two functions enable phones and tablets to provide audio explanation of all functions within the device. You can read non-audio books, text messages and mail, read reminders, set up your contact lists, add new apps, operate apps and adjust the settings systems. There may be some changes to the finger 'tap or swipe' functions as a result of this change, but these are usually explained by the audio itself. Otherwise training courses are recommended.

One important first step is to slow down your hand and finger gestures. Nervousness tends to make you rush things; slow down, a key skill for vision impairment.

The other amazing development for those with vision loss is the growth of voice-activated devices. Just by asking questions the device will respond. Apple products, Elixir (Amazon) and Google Home systems are excellent. For example, you can ask for a cake recipe, information on public transport, the weather, distances and times for travel, how to spell a word, meanings of words, and synonyms and antonyms. Almost any relevant information can be sourced this way.

The other reaction of many people I meet is, 'Oh, I cannot afford it!' or if a little older, 'I can't handle technology!' Both these responses are without validity. Let me deal with the cost factor first.

The Cost Factor

There are many ways to get a smartphone. First, bite the bullet and pay if you can afford it. Many do this through a phone provider. Don't be timid, ask around. Probably the cheapest way to get a smartphone is to ask your family or friends to give you their old phone. Nearly everyone these days has a plan and regularly upgrade to latest models every two years. Don't let their hand-me-down go to children who might well be demanding it, but their needs are not as great as yours. Insist (be assertive) that your needs are to be put first. Being able to function and remain independent are far greater needs and should be prioritised.

Make it clearly known to friends that you really need such a device. There are birthdays, Mother's Days, Father's Days and celebrations of all kinds where your family can contribute to buying the product. The key factor is that you need to know what is best for you. It's always best to examine, feel and experiment first.

For those who might be wondering, the Apple iPhone and computer systems are regarded by totally blind technology experts as having the most accessible and easy to use functions, but the version of the Android system used in Samsung products is apparently 'catching up'.

Some people have asked the Lions Club to assist. Lions have a worldwide vision support foundation, and local clubs are often looking for projects. It doesn't hurt to ask! With the help of someone who knows, you may also be able to access lower cost new products, but be careful about buying off the internet.

In addition, shop around for the best deals for service providers of phone plans. Beware of signing up for vast amounts of download data capacity if you only need the phone for phone contact and organisation. Most people use data for downloading things like movies, and it is unlikely that with vision impairment you will need this facility at the beginning. In any event Netflix has audio-described movies.

You can get a simple phone plan for about A$20 per month, which includes free phone calls.

I Can't Learn or Deal with Technology

'I can't learn!' is the most common response from older people. Assuming cognitive capacity exists, this is no excuse at all! After struggling to use their landline phone and see phone numbers, people well into their 90s have quickly understood the benefits of an audio smartphone once it is explained. They willingly accept training lessons and before long are happy and free again to communicate with friends — and usually for much lower call costs! One woman in her 90s was spending over $400 a month on call costs and was delighted when I explained that, apart from the purchase cost of a new phone and monthly provider costs, calls could be free.

Not only is the habit of trying to 'see' causing intense frustration, but habits are hard to break.

First Steps

The first step is the hardest: what to get and where to go. Most information is accessible by phone. To gain an understanding of what are the cheapest phone providers, discuss with family or friends who they use. It is best to feel and get accustomed to the physical differences before you purchase a phone. Smartphones are very slim and have very few buttons. This tends to alarm those used to large landline phones. Again, if you think a smartphone is too small and you won't be able to see the names or numbers, remember, smartphones can speak to you — you do not need to see or read it!

For more help and information, in Australia, contact blindness agencies Guide Dogs and Vision Australia. Ask for the adaptive technology service, who can discuss phone options and training.

- Vision Australia
- Tel: 1300 84 74 66
- email: athelp@visionaustralia.org

- Guide Dogs
- Tel: 1800 804 805

Be prepared to undertake training in the use of smartphones and as you get used to the finger stroking, tapping and flicking techniques, learn to go slowly!

Other Disability Help Desks

When calling the numbers below, make it clear you have a vision disability.

Apple accessibility hot desk:
- Tel: 1300 365 083
- If you are not disabled, ring: 1300 321 456

Microsoft disability support hot desk
- Tel: 1800 283 300

Google
- Google support is mostly web based, www.google.com.au.
- Tel: 1-866-246-6453
- (Note: Google warns of scams with help or assistance contacts.)

Some Current Best Technology Devices

I've listed some of the latest and best 2021 options below. Keep in mind that as technology is changing so rapidly, these recommendations may be out of date before too long.

Smartphones

These have voice recognition features where you ask a 'digital assistant' to perform functions, for example ask Siri and Ask Google to turn on apps or make calls, text messages, create reminders, or provide information about travel, the weather, and so on. For example, asking Siri 'Where am I?' will give you your location reasonably accurately. You can also spell a word, tell when your next appointment is (ask Siri, 'When is my next appointment, or who is my next appointment with?'), find out the next train, or use notes in your phone to dictate shopping lists.

But importantly, as described above, there are text-to-speech functions such as Voice Over in iPhones and Apple Mac computers as well as Talk Back in Androids where you don't have to see the phone to use it. This voice recognition function is the real breakthrough for those with vision impairment. How many times do you see someone struggling to use their smartphones — 'I can't read texts', 'I can't see the screen!' are typical responses. Putting it bluntly, these responses simply should not be happening.

The Google 'Home' Range

Google 'Home' are voice-activated search and information systems which accesses radio and music. Using Spotify for an additional monthly fee provides almost unlimited access to music. Models are 'Mini', 'Home' and 'Max', obtainable at most tech outlets. The voice-activated systems with 'smart' switches' represent amazing potential for vision impaired people. A range of home systems, including TVs, heaters and lights can work on this system.

There are now smart switches for TV use and central heating. They are, Amazon Firestick $99,Standard or 4K. wifi for Netflicks, plugs into TV and provides voice recognition of commands. For voice activated central heating, Ecobee needs Electrician for re-wiring. You can speak to it for temperature setting.

OrCam

OrCam devices are portable, mounted on glasses, and can read text and convert it to speech using Artificial Intelligence (AI). They also read barcodes and colours, and have special and facial recognition. OrCam is expensive at about A$7,000, but the main advantage is that it is hands-free. Free apps such as seeing AI, for the smartphones can do a similar job.

Some Current Best Apps and Software

Aira Vision

This is a relatively new service based in the USA in which through a smartphone app, professionally trained operators respond to your call in real time and describe what your phone's camera is identifying. You can also buy glasses with a camera attached, making support 'hands free'.

A fee for the Aira service applies. Recently a five-minute free use offer is available, but for those who are eligible, the National

Disability Insurance Scheme (NDIS) will pay for this service. Users report the Aira service is excellent!

Text-to-speech Software for Computers

Some of our best adaptive technology has been invented by people who are blind. For example, Job Access With Speech (JAWS) was designed by Ted Henter along with Bill Joyce in 1987, after Henter had been blinded following a motor accident.

JAWS revolutionised the world of the blind and vision impaired by making any text document, emails, internet sites or documents scanned into the computer, to be read with a synthesised voice. For those with only partial sight loss, screen magnification coupled with changes to screen contrast, or use of a system called Zoom Text, enable computer use. However, if text is made too large, this can make reading tedious and slow so that the employee with vision loss becomes uncompetitive. Contact:

Quantum Technology

Tel: 1300 791 777

www.quantumrlv.com.au

software@quantumr1v.com.au

In 2005, Apple produced its Voice Over software built in to all products without extra cost, and in 1997, Non Visual Desktop Access (NVDA) was designed by Michael Curran and James The, who are both blind. NVDA is available in 48 languages and is not surprisingly, the most popular text-reading software; it is also free. Contact:

Tel: +617 (07) 3149 3306

Website: www.nvda-project.org

Team Viewer

This free software enables access by a remote technology specialist, or friend, to your computer by remote control to assist with solving computer-related problems. This is an essential product where security is protected by a password provided to you, with each access. If you are a JAWS user, there is also an access code for servicing your computer and software remotely.

You could also consider using Microsoft's Quick Assist as an effective alternative for remote access by a technology specialist.

Some More Good Apps

All of the following apps can be downloaded through Apple's App Store or Play Store (for Android). Some outstanding apps include:

For Apple iPhones, Seeing AI — an excellent free text-to-speech reader which also reads barcodes and colours, and features spatial and facial recognition.

For both Android and Apple iOS, the equivalent app to Seeing AI is Supersense AI. This app will read, find objects, and explore places independently, and is free of charge. It provides a set of digital eyes to make the physical world more accessible for the blind. Like Seeing AI, Supersense AI does not need the internet to operate.

An app called Speak! offers similar reading to the two above. It will read any text captured by the camera. It can be used to read anything from street signs to newspapers. The app has been specifically designed to detect text in 'bad photos', for instance when the text is rotated or far away. In addition it knows to detect relevant text only, for example when photographing a page in a book, text captured on the adjacent page will be ignored.

Google Assistant is a voice-activated great information resource similar to Google Home in its capacity to find then read information. It is free. Once installed, ask the assistant to open it, go to approximately the centre of the screen where it announces 'Mike', then tap it twice before asking your question. This is better than Siri as it speaks out most information.

Google Translate for languages is free and excellent.

Aira works through the phone's camera, and involves real people who act as describers. The service is costly, but a free five-minute service is offered.

A free alternative to Aira is Be My Eyes. Supported by volunteers, it does not have the professional readers used by Aira. It is still very good to help you read and identify things.

GPS and public transport apps — their exact titles vary from place to place; for example, in Melbourne, PTV and Tram Tracker or Vline. All are free and excellent for mobility support. Check with your public transport agencies.

For audio books use VA Connect — a free and easy-to-use app that offers access to books, state and regional newspapers, and magazines. Otherwise use the apps available through public libraries, or alternatively Book Share USA, which has an annual fee.

Text-to-speech apps –I recommend Prizmo Go for iPhones or Prizmo for Androids. Voice Dream Scanner for A$10 is a very accurate scanner for reading text. KNFB Reader, which costs about $A160, is very reliable and reads columns.

Cash Reader is excellent for reading all currency notes and costs about A$28 for a lifetime subscription.

There are a number of radio apps, for example in Australia, ABC Listen. If you use Google Home you can access Spotify or any international radio with online services. Also Google and other voice-activated devices will open up radio stations for you.

Supermarket apps — Woolworths, Coles and Aldi have apps, providing the aisle, cost and contents information.

Some Other Apps

- A GPS app called Guide Dogs NSW/ACT, is good and reads overseas maps cost about $28 p.a.
- Use Google Maps, with wifi on and Voice Over on, ask the digital assistant to 'give directions to...' if you are driving, or 'give walking directions to...' and it will speak directions.
- Next There — tells what trains or buses are available from your current location.
- IMove — tells you where you are.
- Wake Me — tells you when your stop is nearby.
- Tap See — can take pictures, read or identify products; it is free.
- Snap Send Solve — an effective app to report mobility-related issues to your local council. Issues include faulty or flooding footpaths, various dangers, etc. It is free, but a little complex to use.
- Metro Notifier — advises of delays with travel.
- Moovit — a O&M recommended free trip planner.

- Transit — bus, train and tram timetables for all capital cities and operating systems; it is free.
- Clew — good for retracing steps in a shopping mall or venue — free.
- Stop Here — for Melbourne, will tell you when a train stop is approaching.
- 1password — for storing your many passwords.
- Colorid — a colour reader.
- Show the Loo — identifies locations of public toilets.

Other Equipment and Gadgets

There are many useful audio or large print (LP) devices that can assist you. Here is a selection:

- Smart TVs — Sony, Samsung and Phillips TVs now have voice recognition features.
- Talking microwave and convection ovens.
- Talking kitchen and bathroom scales. Kitchen scales handle liquid and solids, can be re-set for multiple items, metric or imperial.
- Talking measuring jugs.
- Liquid level sensors with audio alarm for filling cups or other containers, and vibrating model for deafness.
- A personal organiser with adhesive labels called Pen Friend is highly effective for organising your kitchen, pantry, CDs etc.
- Talking thermometers for cooking and health purposes.
- Talking tape measure, with metric and imperial measurements.

- CCTV scanners and optical magnifiers for those with useable sight can be expensive, but funding under a NDIS-provided special technology report is provided.

For low vision:
- Signature guide (small).
- Signature guide (large).
- Envelope address guide.
- A4 superior writing guide.
- Bold line writing pad (A4 & A5).
- Intense black Prokky and Pentil pens — they don't bleed through paper.

For recreation:

- Braille and large print Monopoly, Scrabble, chess, dominos, large print playing cards sets.
- New sports equipment, including basketballs, tennis balls and swish balls with bells in yellow and black.
- Skipping rope which talks the number of skips.

For sewing and handicrafts:

- Infra needle threader (helps thread normal needles).
- Self-thread needles 6 pack.
- Self-thread machine needles.
- Pre-threaded needles pack of 10.
- Reading lamps with magnifiers attached.

Working in the Shed, Mechanics and Other Hobbies

Many people believe that once you have lost sight, you are not able to undertake hobbies, woodwork or mechanics. This is nonsense!

A fear often expressed by partners and family members is that working with power tools and electric saws is too dangerous if you can't see. This is not valid. There are many instances where a partner, in an unwarranted example of over-protection, has demanded that these 'dangerous' tools be sold!' to break the heart of the hobbyist. This attitude arises from a lack of knowledge of what actually can be achieved, a factor most present when sighted people think blindness is associated with helplessness. Yes, care must be taken, but like all independence measures, it is organisation and preparation, setting up jigs, benches and operating systems carefully which makes work safe.

There are many totally blind people making complex furniture such as cupboards, beds, cabinets, chairs and tables, which are vastly superior in quality to any other found on the market. In the process, people who are totally blind are using drop and table saws, lathes, routers and power equipment of all types.

People who are totally blind are remodelling their homes, painting, working on cars, diesel and marine engines and working successfully in garages. One man who is totally blind fully reconditioned and restored a GM Corvette auto.

Marv Ploger, 70, is a blind mechanic in Windorah, south-west of Longreach, Queensland, who worked on cars before his retirement. He jokingly said, 'I've got a 12 by 12 warranty on my work! — driving 12 kilometres, or 12 minutes!' On his retirement after 22 years of blindness he said he has never felt as though he has a disability. 'I didn't know it was a difficulty — I'm just a normal, everyday person,' he said. 'I can pull a motor and gearbox apart, but may need a sighted person to put it back together.'[202]

With the assistance of audio devices it is possible to use large table saws, thicknessers, micrometers and Vernier gauges. There are audio measuring tapes and spirit levels. Even using band saws, lathes and welders are possible. After all, blind people were often sent to protected workshops to make wooden items and mats, but the safety experience of the Assist Program of Vision Australia is that, over 30 years, no serious accident has occurred.

There are totally blind people who successfully maintain their gardens, mow their lawns and trim hedges and trees with electric cutters.

Paul from Melbourne, a Peer and speaker at my discussion groups, says, 'When I work in the garden, I have a radio playing in the garage so that I can orientate myself. I also always place my work tools in a wheelie bin or wheel barrow so that I don't step on them or lose them! I also can service my lawn mower and cut my lawns using my memory or feeling the grass to see what is not cut!'

Another man with limited sight used a series of pegs and string to keep track of how much lawn he had mowed. However, in another case, a man with RP and limited tunnel vision held down the job as gardener in a large factory. His workmates would tease him regularly on the bits of grass he had missed when mowing the lawn. 'Oh!' he cried using the glass half full philosophy, 'But you should see how much I have cut!'

Some Principles for Working with Hobbies, Mechanics or Woodwork

- Be highly organised, think through what you want to do and prepare.
- Go slowly.
- De-clutter your work room and mind.
- Keep things in order, use labellers such as Pen Friend or tactile markers. See also apps and Aira for reading or ID support.
- Keep things simple.
- Standardise tool settings and spacer gauges.
- For woodwork, prepare to spend more time planning and creating your design and jigs, template or measuring guide than making the object itself.
- Use adaptive audio technology.
- For woodwork and metal work — contact the VA Assist Program — Brett Behan, Tel: 03 8378 1225 or 1300 84 74 66.

Some Ideas for Mechanics

The following tips have come from a discussion group of partially sighted and totally blind mechanics who refit and rebuild cars, including electricals, work on differentials, racing cars and maintain go karts, as well as working on trucks, diesel and marine motors, undertake welding and supporting racetrack events. Some of their ideas include:

- Ask for help if you need to, there is no shame in this! There are times when even the most skilful blind mechanics need sighted assistance.

- Don't just place things like spanners on the floor, use a number of plastic tubs to hold screws, bolts, nuts and other small items as well as tools. DO NOT just lay these items down on the ground; it's a guaranteed pathway to stress and frustration.
- Use a checklist (best if you are computer skilled and using text-to-speech software).
- Work on one side of an engine at a time.
- Vernier gauges and micrometers and other equipment such as table saws or thicknessers can be read by a digital audio device to read it. Contact the VA Access Program on Tel: 03 8378 1225.
- Arc welding is like sewing — after 'striking' the rod, move left to right and use guides and gloves.
- At the racetrack — instead of feeling hot engines, ask a sighted person rather than do it yourself.
- Use your hearing to pick up faults.
- Use a radio to hear sound and orientate yourself in a workshop or large area.
- In finding dropped items, use magnets, or a broom to sweep the floor. Don't sweep wildly, sweep in a defined square area.
- Use a dial gauge Vernier with rotating needle.
- Use two torque wrenches pre-set at 35 or 65 pounds or kilos rather than keep adjusting only one wrench.
- Use a 64-piece drill set to act as a measurement check.
- Using feeler gauges for spark plugs set at 2000mm width, place a nick cut into the sheet with the correct gauge thickness.

- Use a talking tape measure (approx. $A190) and if the thickness is less than 10mm use a modified feeler gauge with 1mm blades in a set of 10.
- In centring axles, use a slider gauge.
- To assist depth measurement, make up shims at different sizes.
- Most mechanical work is repetitive and a good memory is essential.
- Replacing tyres — use thin aluminium or stainless steel tubes to place over the thread and thus extend wheel studs, or use a jack using fingers to align studs.
- A Super Chief jack for tyres costs about $A30.
- When working with electrical wiring, use a standard multimeter — from Repco or a colour detector such as the colour detector app for iPhones.
- Use an audio liquid level measure to test quantity of oils, petrol (but don't use the one in your kitchen!).
- Use a barcode reader to identify oils and other liquids.
- For hard concrete surfaces, use a special foam rubber mat.
- For replacing parts for engines which are out of stock or no longer made, contact a special machine shop.

Some Audio and Vision Impaired Adjusted Tools

- Talking tape measure.
- Audio speakers for Vernier gauges or table saws — contact the VA Assist Program — Brett Behan, Tel: 03 8378 1225 or 1300 84 74 66.
- Audio liquid level measure — contact VA, Tel: 1300 84 74 66.

- Audio spirit levels.
- Click Rule — a simple gauge with extensions in 1mm or 10 mm increments slides out — excellent low cost option for micro measurements.
- Wipe on Poly from Feast Watson — an easy to use polyurethane timber finish.
- You can make a cheap device to measure the centre of a dowel — create a perfect 45-degree right angle and then glue a piece of wood exactly on the 45-degree cut line to project into the middle of the set square. Running two cross lines along this will provide the exact centre.

CONCLUSION

In coming to the end of this book, I sincerely hope that it has inspired you to take action while also contributing to your knowledge of vision loss. That , while loss of vision is naturally difficult if not frightening at first, vision loss is something we can adjust to and change the way we think about this disability and how we can change and adjust. I hope it has helped you to understand that vision loss and blindness are not the end of a life, but a beginning for a new one.

Learning to do things differently can be immensely empowering and accepting our disability is a strength, not weakness. If, in reading this book you feel empowered to take action, telephone a blindness and vision impaired service agency to initiate support and training. I provide a summary list of Agencies in Appendix One which you might be able to find on the Internet. The first step for action — to pick up a phone. Join a peer groups, reskill yourself and begin to use latest technology, then this book will have accomplished its primary objective. If as an onlooker to vision loss, it has increased your knowledge and understanding of this complex subject, then another important objective has been realised.

Cameron D. Algie 2021

Contacting The Author

Cameron can be contacted on his web site, - 'I Can See Clearly Books, Seeing Things Differently' on:

www.icanseeclearly books.com

APPENDIX

A Summary of Australian and International Service Organisations

List Of International Blindness Organisations

Contacts for the following can be found on the Internet.

- Action for Blind People (UK)
- American Council of the Blind
- American Foundation for the Blind - a site containing
  - American Printing House for the Blind
  - Blind World - an online magazine for the blind and vision impaired.
  - Blindness Resource Center - contains many links to blindness related websites.
- Bookshare - an international library available to people with print reading disabilities and/or vision impairments in over 36 countries.
- Canadian National Institute for the Blind

- EnableLink.com - the online community for people who are blind or vision impaired, their families, friends
- Equipment for Kenya
- Hadley School for the Blind
- Library of Congress (USA)
- National Federation of the Blind (USA)
- National Federation of the Blind: Advocates for Equality (Canada)
- Royal National Institute for the Blind (UK)
- Royal New Zealand Foundation of the Blind
- Vision Australia
- World Blind Union

AUSTRALIA (Principal bodies)

- Blind Citizens Australia
  National
  www.bca.org.au

- Blind Cricket Australia
  National
  www.blindcricket.org.au

- Blind Golf Australia National
  www.blindgolf.com.au

- Blind Sailing Australia
  National
  www.blindsportsaustralia.com.au/sailing-

- Blind Sports & Recreation Victoria
  Victoria
  www.blindsports.org.au

- Blind Sports Australia
  National
  www.blindsportsaustralia.com.au 2,600

- Braille House (Australia)   National
  www.braillehouse.org.au

- Charles Bonnet Syndrome Foundation   National

- Guide Dogs Australia
   National
  guidedogs.com.au
  Also, Guide Dogs in NSW, Vic, Qld, Tas &WA

- Queensland blind association
  Queensland
  qldblind.org.au
  Peer

- Royal Institute of deaf blind Children
  National
  www.rdbc.org.au
  Royal Institute of deaf blind Children
  National
  www.rdbc.org.au

- Royal Society for the blind National
  www.rsb.org.au

- South Pacific Education in Vision Impairment   National
  www.spevi.net
  Statewide Vision Resource Center (Vic) Victoria
  www,svrc.vic.edu.au

- Vision 2020 Australia
  National
  www.vision2020australia.org.au/ 42

- Vision Australia (VA)
  National
  www.visionaustralia.org

- VA Library and Feelix Library O&M and Employment services

Endnotes

1   Poulson, Jane, The Doctor Will Not See You Now, Novalis Publications, 2001. Dr Poulson was the first blind doctor to be admitted to practise in Canada.

2   Erik Weihenmayer, Touch The Top of the World, Plume Books, 2001. Weihenmayer is a bestselling author, athlete, adventurer, and motivational speaker. He is the only blind person to reach the summit of Mount Everest. He also completed the Seven Summits, joining 150 mountaineers who have accomplished that feat, but the only climber who was blind with retinoschisis, a retinal disease where layers of the retina separated, eventually losing sight with glaucoma.

3   'If' by Rudyard Kipling.

4   American Foundation for the Blind (AFB) research 2018.

5   Lebers optic amorosis is an inherited condition affecting the retina.

6   Maribel Steel, Blindness for Beginners, self-published, 2019, p.83.

7   Psychologist Christopher Hall Maps, Director, Australian Centre for Grief and Bereavement, 'Beyond Kübler-Ross: Recent developments in our understanding of grief and bereavement,' InPsych 2011, Vol. 33, December, Issue 6.

8   Too much quinine causes ocular quinine toxicity producing symptoms of blurred/loss of vision, defective colour vision, and constricted visual field. (See the British Journal of Ophthalmology, 29 September 2020. Bbjo.bmj.com)

9   Dr Colin Murray Parkes, consultant psychiatrist, Australian Centre for Grief and Bereavement, 2019.

10 Maps, Professor Christopher Hall, Director, Australian Centre for Grief and Bereavement, 'Beyond Kübler-Ross: Recent developments in our understanding of grief and bereavement,' InPsych 2011 | Vol 33 December | Issue 6.

11 BBC, 'Blindness and Mental Health Can Come Hand in Hand', 26 March 2019.

12 McCallum, Professor Ron, Born at the Right Time, Allen & Unwin, Sydney, 2019

13 Dr Rob Gordon, clinical psychologist, has worked in the field of disaster recovery since Ash Wednesday in 1983. He is a consultant to the Red Cross and the Victorian Department of Health and Human Services; see Better Health Channel.

14 ABC radio, 20 January 2020.

15 Sherri S. Tepper, The Visitor, Harper Voyager, 2009.

16   Hugh Mackay, psychologist and social researcher, ABC RN, 'Life Matters', 11 August 2020

17   Leigh Sales, Any Ordinary Day, Penguin Books Australia, 2018.

18   Refractive errors are near-sightedness (myopia), far-sightedness (hyperopia) and astigmatism (presbyopia). The most common symptom is blurred vision, diagnosed by eye examination. Treatment options are glasses, contact lenses or surgery. Source: US National Eye Institute, 31 Center Drive MSC 2510, Bethesda, MD 20892.

19   Hugh R. Taylor, Jill E. Keeffe, Hien T. V. Vu, Jie Jin Wang, Elena Rochtchina, Paul Mitchell and M. Lynne Pezzullo, 'Vision Loss in Australia', Medical Journal of Australia, 2005, 182 (11), and American Macular Degeneration Foundation (AMDF) https://www.macular.org, accessed 2019.

20   Medline Plus, USA 2008 issue, vol. 3, no 3, pp. 14, 15.

21   Ruanne Vent-Schmidt PhD, Canadian National Institute for the Blind (CNIB), Vancouver, October 2019.

22   Australian Government, Department of Health, 2008.

23   American Foundation for the Blind (AFB), Glossary of Eye Conditions, 2018.

24   A person is considered legally blind if they cannot see at 6 metres what someone with normal vision can see at 60 metres, or if their field of vision is less than 20 degrees. Source: Vision Australia, https://www.visionaustralia.org.

25   National Eye Institute (NEI), USA, and Commonwealth Department of Health report, 2008.

26   For an excellent description of an operation to remove a tumour on the optic nerve, see Henry Marsh, Do No Harm: Stories of Life, Death and Brain Surgery, Weidenfeld & Nicolson, London, 2014, chapter 4.

27   National Centre for Biotechnology Information, US National Library of Medicine, Bethesda, Maryland. Writers, Trevor Huff and Scott C. Dulebohn, 2018.

28   Ron McCallum, Born at the Right Time, Allen & Unwin, Sydney, 2019.

29   If 18 per cent of those with severe sight loss, but not totally blind, are considered.

30   Doidge, N. The Brain That Changes itself, Stories of personal triumph. Pub.2007, Viking Press

31   Chris Plummer, Neurologist, ABC RN, 'All in The Mind', 2 August 2020.

32   Canadian National Blind Foundation NIB Foundation, Vision Australia and the Blind Foundation of New Zealand, 16 November 2018.

33   Jane Poulson, The Doctor Will Not See You Now, Novalis Publications, 2001.

34   Mary Bates, 'Super Powers for the Blind and Deaf', Scientific American, May 2012, scientificamerican.com.

35   François Champoux, director of the University of Montreal's Laboratory in the functional neuroimaging unit (UNF), 8 May 2012.

36   Corinna Bauer, 'Neuro Plasticity and Blind People', Journal of Public Library Of Science, 23 March 2017.

37   Thomas Politzer, O.D. Former NORA President, Neuro-Optometric Rehabilitation Association, Brainline.org, 2019.

38   Neuro-Optometric Rehabilitation Association (NORA), https://noravisionrehab.com/-vision.

39   Dr Corinna Bauer, the Schepens Eye Research Institute of Massachusetts Eye and Ear Hospital as reported in PLOS one, 23 March 2017.

40   WHO, World Report on Eye Health, 8 October 2019.

41   Seth Flaxman and Rupert Bourne, 'Global Causes of Blindness and Distance Vision Impairment 1990–2020: A Systematic Review and Meta-Analysis', The Lancet Global Health, Vol. 5, issue 12.

42   The Lancet Global Health, lead author, Prof Rupert Bourne, from Anglia Ruskin University, and BBC News, 2 August 2017.

43   Night blindness, a type of vision impairment also known as nyctalopia, means poor vision at night or in dimly lit environments, or changing from a well-lit area to dark. It doesn't mean you can't see, but it can be caused by myopia, cataracts, retinitis pigmentosa, Usher's Syndrome, pancreatic insufficiency, high blood sugar or diabetes, or in rare cases lack of Vitamin A (retinol).

44   Michelle Hackman, 'Why Do People Fear the Blind?', AFB, 1 June 2014, https://www.afb.org/blog/entry/why-do-people-fear-blind#:~:text=Blindness%20is%20not%20a%20life,akin%20to%20losing%20life%2C%20altogether.

45   Professor Ron McCallum, Born at the Right Time, Allen & Unwin, 2019.

46   Steve Kelley, 'I'm Not Blind', American Foundation for the Blind (AMFB), 2016, https://visionaware.org/blog/visually-impaired-now-what/im-not-blind/.

47   Haben Girma (born July 29, 1988) is an American disability rights advocate, and the first deafblind graduate of Harvard Law School.

48   Erik Weihenmayer has written three books: No Barriers: A Blind Man's Journey to Kayak the Grand Canyon, St Martin's Press, 2017; Touch the Top of the World, Plume Books, 2001; and The Adversity Advantage: Turning Everyday Struggles Into Everyday Greatness, Fireside, 2007.

49   Michael Hingson, Thunder Dog, Thomas Nelson, 2012.

50   As told to the author in a talk to Vision Australia Peers in 2012.

51   Janet won a bronze medal in the 2004 Paralympics and silver and bronze in the World IPC Championships in 2002.

52   The Australian Women's Weekly, 1 May 2018.

53   Michael Hingson, Thunder Dog, Thomas Nelson, 2012.

54   Innes G. Finding A Way, Pub. 2016, University of Queensland Press. Graeme Innes AM, was Australia's Disability Discrimination Commissioner from December 2005 to July 2014. A human rights advocate for the past 30 years he has played a role in many human rights and disability initiatives, including drafting of the United Nations Convention on the Rights of Persons with Disabilities. His AM awarded in recognition of his human rights work and his contribution to the rights of people with disability.

55   Joy Thomas, writer and teacher with RP, writing for Vision Aware, American Foundation for the Blind, 2018.

56   Poll conducted by Alliance for Eye and Vision Research (AEVR) USA, in 2014.

57   Dr Adrienne Scott, assistant professor of ophthalmology at Johns Hopkins University School of Medicine, Baltimore, 2016.

58   Rosemary Mahoney, 'Why Do We Fear the Blind?', New York Times, 2016.

59   Joy Thomas, writing for Vision Aware, American Foundation for the Blind, 2018.

60   Erik Weihenmayer, Touch the Top of the World, Plume Books, 2001.

61   Barbara Cheadle, 'My Body Belongs To Me,' NOPBS conference and NFB News article, 2019

62   Chicago Lighthouse Foundation, USA, 2018.

63   Innes G. Finding A Way, Pub. 2016, University of Queensland Press.

64   Maribel Steel, Blindness for Beginners, self-published, 2019, p.12.

65   Vision Australia's Feelix Library has a world-class service of tactile books for vision-impaired children, as well as audio books for children. There is also a large audio library for adults.

66   Erik Weihenmayer, Touch the Top of the World, Plume Books, 2001.

67   Dianne Ashworth, I Spy With My Bionic Eye, self-published, 2017.

68   Ali Gripper, The Barefoot Surgeon, Allen & Unwin, 2018, chapter 2.

69   Research by Dr Lisel Dwyer, Flinders University, November 2014.

70   'Women Outperform Men in 11 of 12 Key Emotional Intelligence Competencies', Los Angeles, 7 March 2016 — research by the Korn Ferry division of Korn Ferry (NYSE: KFY); women score higher than men on nearly all emotional intelligence competencies.

71   Australia, telephone conference for dog guide users, 6 April 2019.

72   Sarah Jenkins, 'People Think You Can't Be Blind and Use a Phone', BBC News, 29 January 2019.

73   David W. Johnson, Reaching Out, Interpersonal Effectiveness and Self-Actualization (with reference to Carl Rogers), 11th Edition, 2014.

74   Women normally represent over 70 per cent of group participants.

75   Psychologist Christine Bagley Jones, Qld, ABC Radio, 9 August 2020.

76   Dr Martin Seligman, psychologist, Learned Optimism, Vintage, 2006 (First Pub, 1990). Selegman is a leading proponent of the concept of Positive Psychology, and author of many books, including The Hope Circuit: A Psychologist's Journey from Helplessness to Optimism, 2014.

77   Professor Christopher Peterson, A Primer in Positive Psychology, OUP, 2006.

78   Professor Lea Asher, ABC Radio, Monday, 3 August 2019.

79   Eve Waters, Psychologist, ABC Radio, Saturday, 6 July 2019.

80   Interview with Anne Leadbetter, ABC Radio, Wednesday, 6 February 2019.

81   Dr Rob Gordon, clinical psychologist, works in the field of disaster recovery since Ash Wednesday in 1983. He is a consultant to the Red Cross and the Victorian Department of Health and Human Services; see Better Health Channel.

82   Dr William Worden, Grief Counseling and Grief Therapy, 4th ed., New York, 2008.

83   Dr Colin Murray Parkes, OBE, MD, Forsyth, DL. consultant psychiatrist, Australian Centre for Grief and Bereavement.

84   Fifty per cent of participants in Quality Living Groups reported failure of professionals to refer them on to rehabilitative support services, although this was trending upwards by 2019.

85   Dr Stephanie Dowrick, psychologist, The Age, 2007.

86   Sheila Hocken, Emma and I, Dutton Books, 1978, chapter 5.

87   'I Have a Dream' speech, August 1963.

88   Leigh Sales, Any Ordinary Day, Penguin, 2019.

89   Maribel Steel, Blindness For Beginners, self-published, 2019.

90   Sally Capp, ABC Radio, 9 March 2019.

91   As discussed by Carl Sagan in his book, The Dragons of Eden, 1977, the American physician and neuroscientist Paul D. MacLean proposed the 'Reptilian' brain theory. Known as the triune brain it consists of the reptilian complex, the paleomammalian complex (limbic system), and the neomammalian complex (neocortex), viewed each as independently conscious, and as structures sequentially added to the forebrain in the course of evolution. However, this hypothesis has been subject to criticism, and is no longer espoused by the majority of comparative neuroscientists.

92   'What is the science behind fear?', CNN News, 29 October 2015, https://edition.cnn.com/2015/10/29/health/science-of-fear/index.html, and https://www.theskysthelimitconsulting.com

93   L. Saulsman, P. Nathan, L. Lim and H. Correia, What? Me Worry!?! Mastering Your Worries, Module 11, Centre for Clinical Interventions, Perth, Western Australia. ISBN: 0-9751985-9-9 January, 2005.

94   Centre For Clinical Intervention, WA Government Department of Health.

95   Hugh Mackay, psychologist and social researcher, speaking on ABC RN, Life Matters, 11 August 2020

96   www.mayoclinic.org, 17 August 2018.

97   headspace.org.au. The Headspace app is available on the App Store and Google Play.

98   Alvin Powell, 'When Science Meets Mindfulnesss', 9 April 2018, and Leslie Ripel, 'Mindfulness and the Brain', 11 September 2020, positivepsychology.com.

99   'Mindfulness Meditation Training Alters How We Process Fearful Memories', EurekAlert, 15 October 2015, https://www.eurekalert.org/pub_releases/2019-10/mgh-mmt101519.php.

100   Beyond Blue (Australia), www.beyoundblue.org.

101   Caroline Steber, '11 Early Signs of Depression to Have on Your Radar', Bustle, 26 July 2019.

102   Austroads, 'Assessing Fitness to Drive', austroads.com.au.

103   Inability to recognise faces is one of the most frequently raised concerns in discussion groups.

104   '22 Facts about the Brain', www.dentinstitute.com.

105   Nikhil Swaminathan on 29 April 2008 quoting study by the National Academy of Sciences USA.

106   For detailed information, see https://www.bca.org.au/toolkits/.

107   Erik Weihenmayer, Touch the Top of the World, Plume Books, 2001.

108   Heidi in conversations with the author, 2015.

109   Steve Kelley, 'I'm Not Blind', Low Vision Tech, 2016, https://www.lowvisiontech.com/im-not-blind/.

110   Erik Weihenmayer, Touch the Top of the World, Plume Books, 2001.

111   F. Ozbay et al., 'Social Support and Resilience to Stress', Psychiatry, May 2007, http://www.ncbi.nlm.nih.gov/pmc/articles/PMC2921311/

112   Client responses to the author's discussion groups 2007-19.

113   www.ourconsumerplace.com.au; Wikipedia, https://www.socialworkhelper.com.

114   Dr Hugh Mackay, ABC RN Life Matters, 11 August 2020.

115   Jane Poulson, The Doctor Will Not See You Now, Novalis Publications, 2001.

116   Sir David Fletcher Jones, entrepreneur and pioneer of workplace participation.

117 Michael Hingson, Thunder Dog, Thomas Nelson, 2011.

118 Samantha Gash, Australian ultra-marathon runner, ABC Radio, 12 September 2020.

119 Rohit Roy, Melbourne man on ABC Radio Melbourne, Drive Program, 15 September 2020, on how he gave up 'fizzy drinks'.

120 In 1831, in Boston, Samuel Gridley Howe, founded the first school for the blind, which with the Perkins school, commenced the modern belief that people with vision loss could become independent and employable.

In the late 1800s special Institutions for the blind were established in Australia: the New South Wales Institution for the Deaf, Dumb and Blind in 1869, a similar organisation in South Australia (1874) and others such as the Royal Victorian Institute for the Blind (RVIB) in 1891, with a school at St Kilda Road and later at Burwood in Victoria. St Paul's School for the Blind in Kew offered specialised education for young children, and a Braille Library in Victoria was established in 1903.

121 Jane Poulson, The Doctor Will Not See You Now, Novalis Publishing, Toronto, 2001.

122 Janet Shaw, Beyond the Red Door, Boolarong Press, 2012.

123 Janet Shaw, ibid.

124 Janet Shaw, ibid.

125 Opening Eyes onto Inclusion and Diversity, Melissa Cain and Melissa Fanshawe, p.8. University of Southern Queensland, https://usq.pressbooks.pub/openingeyes/chapter/%e2%80%a2opening-eyes-to-vision-impairment-inclusion-is-just-another-way-of-seeing/

126 Department of Social Services, Australian Government — Shut Out: The Experience of People with Disabilities and their Families in Australia, 1 May 2012.

127 Media Access Australia, co-author CEO, Alex Varley, October 2013.

128 Lawrie McCredie's discussions with the author 1976.

129 The CNIB Foundation, Vision Australia and the Blind Foundation of New Zealand, 16 November 2018.

130 Blind Citizens Australia (BCA) News, June 2019.

131 Norman Doidge MD, The Brain That Changes itself, 2007; and The Brain's Way of Healing, 2015.

132 Erik Weihenmayer, Touch the Top of the World, Plume Books, 2001, chapter 8.

133 Lawrie McCredie in discussions with the author, 1976.

134 The CNIB Foundation, Vision Australia and the Blind Foundation of New Zealand, 16 November 2018.

135 Disability Statistics Resources, Australian Network on Disability, https://www.and.org.au/pages/disability-statistics.html. Also: Australian Institute of Health and Welfare, https://www.aihw.gov.au/getmedia/f732bc12-1787 ... /Employment-20906.pdf.asp.

136 Blind Citizens Australia (BCA), News, June 2019.

137 Australian Human Rights Commission, Face the Facts: Disability Rights, 25 February 2015.

138 Sandra Budd, CRNIB, VA, BFNZ research paper, Nov. 2018.

139 The CNIB Foundation, Vision Australia and the Blind Foundation of New Zealand, 16 November 2018.

140 Innes G.Finding a Way Pub. 2016 Queensland University Press.

141 Department of Social Services, Australia, Shut Out, https://www.dss.gov.au/our-responsibilities/disability-and-carers/publications-articles/policy-research/shut-out-the-experience-of-people-with-disabilities-and-their-families-in-australia, 7 November 2014.

142 Victorian Parliament, inquiry into Social Inclusion and Victorians with Disabilities, 2014.

143 'To Face the Future of Work, We Need New Approaches', BCA News, June 2019, www.bca.org.au.

144 Barbara Pierce, Editor, The Braille Monitor, member, Committee on the Status of Blind Women, World Blind Union, 1999, www.nfb.org. Speech to the 1997 NFB National Convention in July.

145 Barbara Pierce, Editor, The Braille Monitor, member, Committee on the Status of Blind Women, World Blind Union, 1999, www.nfb.org.

146 Young Blind Citizens Australia (YBCA), 'Blind Living: Hair, Beauty and Fashion', 2019, www.bca.com.org/ybcv or request contact information for the YBCV committee from the head BCA office, Tel: 03 9654 1400, 1800 033 660.

147 Erik Weihenmayer, Touch the Top of the World, Plume Books, 2001.

148 Sara Taylor, 'Five Dating Tips for People who Are Blind or Have Low Vision', Vision Australia, Community News, 3 February 2020.

149 Erik Weihenmayer, Touch the Top of the World, Plume Books, 2001.

150 Australia's Gender Pay Gap Statistics, 17 August 2020, WGEA, www.wgea.gov.au.

151 Pew Research Center, https://www.pewresearch.org/fact-tank/2019/03/22/gender-pay-gap-facts/.

152 BBC News, 'Gender Pay Gap: Men Still Earn More Than Women at Most Firms', 21 February 2018, https://www.bbc.com/news/business-43129339.

153 Online survey, 8–21 August and 14–28 September 2017, using Pew Research Center's American Trends Panel.

154 Erik Weihenmayer, Touch the Top of the World, Plume Books, 2001.

155 Graeme Innes, blind former Equal Opportunity Disability Commissioner, discussions with the author 2015.

156 L. Penny Rosenblum, Sunggye Hong, Beth Harris, 'Experiences of Parents with Visual Impairments Who Are Raising Children', Journal of Visual Impairment & Blindness, vol. 103, no. 2, February 2009.

157 Victoria, blind parent talk to parents and author, 2015.

158 Heidi, in talks with the author in 2015.

159 L. Penny Rosenblum, Sunggye Hong, Beth Harris, 'Experiences of Parents with Visual Impairments Who Are Raising Children', Journal of Visual Impairment & Blindness, vol. 103, no. 2, February 2009.

160 Megan Sety, 'The Impact of Domestic Violence on Children: A Literature Review', Benevolent Society, 2016.

161 Personal Safety Survey, Australian Bureau of Statistics, 2006.

162 Maribel Steel, Blindness for Beginners, self-published, 2019, p.17.

163 Maribel Steel, Blindness For Beginners, self-published 2019, pp.17–35.

164 University of Michigan Genetics consent protocol, 2019.

165 Prenatal diagnostic testing is used to detect changes in a foetus's genes or chromosomes. This type of testing is offered to couples with an increased risk of having a baby with a genetic or chromosomal disorder. A tissue sample for testing can be obtained through amniocentesis or chorionic villus sampling. US National Library of Medicine.

166 Sheila Hocken, Emma and I, Dutton Books, 1978.

167 L. Penny Rosenblum, Sunggye Hong, Beth Harris, 'Experiences of Parents with Visual Impairments Who Are Raising Children', Journal of Visual Impairment & Blindness, vol. 103, no. 2, February 2009.

168 McCallum,Professor Ron, Born at the Right Time, Allen & Unwin, 2019.

169 Geoff Bowen, 'Misconceptions About Visual Impairment', Psychologist State-wide Vision Resource Centre, Victoria, 2019.

170 Barbara Pierce, 'The Blind Child, Part of the Family, Part of the World', National Federation for the Blind, USA, 2019, https://www.nfb.org//images/nfb/publications/fr/fr21/fr06ws18.htm.

171 Barbara Pierce, ibid.

172 Barbara Pierce, Editor, The Braille Monitor, member, Committee on the Status of Blind Women, World Blind Union.1999 www.nfb.org.

173 As reported to the author by Margaret Fialides, Manager, Tape Reading Service, RVIB, July, 2019.

174 Post Traumatic Stress Syndrome is 'Readily defined as symptoms consistent with posttraumatic stress disorder (PTSD), but that occur earlier than 30 days after experiencing the traumatic event, posttraumatic stress syndrome (PTSS) is now acknowledged to be a serious health issue.' Stephen Sparks, 'Posttraumatic Stress Syndrome, What Is it?', Journal of Trauma Nursing, 2018, vol. 25, no. 1.

175 Geoff Bowen, 'Misconceptions about Visual Impairment', Psychologist, Statewide Vision Resource Centre, Victoria, 2019.

176 medlineplus.gov, Medical Encyclopedia; also Jane Wakefield, BBC Technology, 27 March 2015, https://www.bbc.com/news/technology-32067158.

177 Geoff Bowen, 'Misconceptions about Visual Impairment', Psychologist, Statewide Vision Resource Centre, Victoria, 2019.

178 Learning Disabilities and Visual Impairments Workshop Assessment of Learning Disabilities In Students with Visual Impairment, Texas School for the Blind.

179 Keratoconus is a progressive eye disease causing a thinning of the clear front surface of the eye (cornea) and distorts the cornea into a cone-like shape. Keratoconus cannot be corrected with spectacles and may be caused by an imbalance of enzymes. It causes myopia, glare, and distorted and blurred vision. Corneal transplants are possible. Source: Dr William Trattler, Ophthalmologist, https://www.allaboutvision.com/en-au/conditions/keratoconus/.

180 Learning Disabilities and Visual Impairments Workshop Assessment of Learning Disabilities in Students with Visual Impairment, Texas School for the Blind.

181 Penny L. Rosenblum, Sunggye Hong and Beth Harris, 'Experiences of Parents with Visual Impairments Who Are Raising Children', Journal of Visual Impairment & Blindness, Vol. 103, No. 2, Feb. 2009.

182 Barbara Pierce, 'The Blind Child, Part of the Family, Part of the World', National Federation of the Blind (NFVB).

183 Lori A. Roggman, Lisa K. Boyce and Mark S. Innocenti, Developmental Parenting: A Guide for Early Childhood Practitioners, Brookes Publishing, Maryland, 2008.

184 Melissa Cain and Melissa Fanshawe, 'Opening Eyes onto Inclusion and Diversity', University of Southern Queensland, https://usq.pressbooks.pub/openingeyes.

185 Hocken ,Sheila, Emma and I, Dutton Books, 1978.

186 Janet Shaw, Beyond the Red Door, Boolarong Press, 2012.

187 The National Association for the Education of Young Children; Lori A. Roggman, Lisa K. Boyce and Mark S. Innocenti, Developmental Parenting: A Guide for Early Childhood Practitioners, Brookes Publishing, Maryland, 2008.

188 Productivity Commission, Housing Decisions of Older Australians, 2015, figure 11.

189 Jane Poulson, The Doctor Will Not See You Now, Novalis Publications, 2001.

190 Jane Poulson, ibid.

191 Jane Poulson, ibid.

192 Blind Alliance Newsletter, November 2019, sourced from 'Girl Gone Blind Registered' Blog, 14 June 2015.

193 Barbara Pierce, Editor, The Braille Monitor, 'Love, Dating, and Marriage: Blind Children Grow Up and Become Parents, Too', Future Reflections, Vol. 7, No. 1; 'Reflections on the Importance of Socialization for Blind Girls and Women', Future Reflections, Vol. 16, No. 4, https://www.nfb.org.

194 From Blind Alliance Newsletter, November 2019, sourced from 'Girl Gone Blind Registered' Blog 14 June 2015.

195 Australian Bureau of Statistics, 2006, 2017.

196 Australian Network on Disability resources, 2018, https://www.and.org.au/pages/disability-statistics.html.

197 Face the Facts, 2018, Disability Statistics Resources and Australian Network on Disability Resources, 2018, https://www.and.org.au/pages/disability-statistics.html.

198 US Bureau of Justice Statistics 2009–2014 (BJS) as reported by Audrey Demmitt, RN, Vision Aware peer advisor, 2018.

199 Australian Human Rights Commission, Equal Before the Law, 2014, https://humanrights.gov.au/our-work/disability-rights/publications/equal-law.

200 Leigh Canet, Defensive Concepts Australia, 2019.

201 Disability Statistics Resources, Australian Network on Disability, https://www.and.org.au/pages/disability-statistics.html.

202 ABC television documentary, 2017.

www.ingramcontent.com/pod-product-compliance
Lightning Source LLC
Chambersburg PA
CBHW021848020426
42334CB00013B/238